1,001 Tips for Living Well with Diabetes

"Diabetes touches every community, and has particularly ravaged the American Indian community, with approximately 15 percent of American Indians and Native Alaskans receiving care for the disease. The key to managing diabetes is knowledge, and *1,001 Tips for Living Well with Diabetes* offers just that. McQuown's book is a must read for anyone looking for a way to better cope with this disease."

—SENATOR BEN NIGHTHORSE CAMPBELL (Colorado), Senate Diabetes Caucus

■

"This fine book by Judith H. McQuown, *1,001 Tips for Living Well with Diabetes,* written from the patient's point of view, provides a much-needed aid for successful coping with this disease. The book is written as a compendium of a huge volume of practical information. Fortunately, it has been cleverly designed, so that it can be read in part, in whole, or skipping around from section to section. This novel approach to a diabetes manual provides easy access for everyone. It should occupy a prominent spot on the bookshelf of every diabetic individual. It should also be of great use to physicians trying to cope with assisting their patients in living well with the disease."

—EDWARD MERKER, MD, FACE, Chief, Endocrinology, Diabetes and Metabolism, Cabrini Medical Center, Associate Clinical Professor of Medicine and Geriatrics, Mount Sinai School of Medicine

■

"Just when you think you know everything (well, almost everything), out comes a book like *1,001 Tips for Living Well with Diabetes*. Just turn to any page and you're sure to discover a new, creative way to make living with diabetes just a little bit easier."

—GARY SCHEINER, MS, CDE, author of *Think Like a Pancreas: A Practical Guide to Managing Diabetes with Insulin*

"*1,001 Tips for Living Well with Diabetes* is a reader-friendly and practical guide to coping with what has rapidly become a major national and international health crisis. Those struggling with the worldwide pandemic of diabetes—as well as their friends and families—can gain valuable insights on how to cope with the disease and improve their quality of life by applying the common-sense lessons offered by Judith McQuown in this eminently readable how-to guide."
—CONGRESSWOMAN CAROLYN B. MALONEY (New York)

"Judith's book is a terrific compendium of easy, do-it-yourself measures to reverse this deadly disease—or at least to minimize its debilitating effects. Each idea is so concisely and compellingly written that you can't help but keep reading for more."
—MARJORY ABRAMS, Publisher, Boardroom, Inc.

"Well done! Rather than focusing on surviving diabetes, Judith McQuown inspires us to thrive—in spite of diabetes. She knows—from life experience—that diabetes is more than a medical condition; rather it affects our emotional and spiritual as well as physical selves. Her tips speak to all aspects of life with diabetes—something sorely needed for people like us who continue to live with this condition each day."
—GABRIELLE KAPLAN-MAYER, author of *Insulin Pump Therapy Demystified* (www.insulinpumpbook.com)

"I would recommend this book to anyone with diabetes. The information McQuown provides is comprehensive, practical, and easy to read. Through this book, diabetics will be better informed about nutrition, exercise, medications, and other important aspects of living with this disease. . . . A book that will benefit many diabetics and their loved ones."
—GIFFORD MILLER, Speaker of The Council of The City of New York

"Diabetics . . . with pain, weakness, fatigue, and other impairments . . . will find this book very helpful. Throughout the book and especially in the chapter on exercise, Ms. McQuown provides many tips and useful words of encouragement that can help individuals start and maintain their exercise programs and activities that promote movement. . . . The practical and sometimes humorous style of Ms. McQuown's writing makes it a pleasure to read and makes it easier for individuals to achieve those goals. I highly recommend this book for diabetics."
—ALAN P. MIRASOL, MD, Department of Physical Medicine and Rehabilitation, Lenox Hill Hospital

1,001 Tips *for* Living Well *with* Diabetes

1,001
Tips *for* Living Well *with* Diabetes

FIRSTHAND ADVICE THAT REALLY WORKS

■ Judith H. McQuown ■

Foreword by Harry Gruenspan, MD, PhD

MARLOWE & COMPANY
NEW YORK

AVALON

Library of Congress Cataloging-in-Publication Data is available.

ISBN 1-56924-435-9

9 8 7 6 5 4 3 2 1

Designed by Pauline Neuwirth, Neuwirth & Associates, Inc.
Printed in the United States of America
Distributed by Publishers Group West

Every area of trouble gives out a ray of hope, and the one unchange-able certainty is that nothing is certain or unchangeable.

—JOHN F. KENNEDY

What would life be if we had no courage to attempt anything?

—VINCENT VAN GOGH

When you're going through hell, keep going.

—WINSTON CHURCHILL

For

Harold Allen Lightman

Contents

CONTENTS

CONTENTS

CONTENTS

CONTENTS

CONTENTS

CONTENTS

CONTENTS

3: Working with Your Doctors and Other Health-Care Professionals

CONTENTS

CONTENTS

CONTENTS

CONTENTS

CONTENTS

CONTENTS

CONTENTS

CONTENTS

CONTENTS

CONTENTS

CONTENTS

CONTENTS

CONTENTS

CONTENTS

CONTENTS

Foreword

by Harry Gruenspan, MD, PhD

DIABETES RATES ARE predicted to double worldwide to 366 million people by the year 2030. The incidence of the disease is increasing precipitously throughout the world. No country is being spared. The rate of increase in poorer countries is even steeper than in developed ones. Adult onset diabetes is caused by a genetic predisposition expressed in modern social circumstances. The luxury of inactivity and the abundance of calories produced by technological advance conspire to cause disease in the predisposed. Diabetes is the leading cause of blindness in the United States. It is also the leading cause of kidney disease and amputations. There is an inordinate toll attributable to heart disease and stroke. In 2002, direct and indirect costs of diabetes in the United States were estimated at $132 billion; 186,000 people died of diabetes in that year, mostly due to the cardiovascular complications of diabetes. It is critical that human toll and financial burden of the disease be reduced.

It is possible to prevent and delay the complications of diabetes. Tight control of blood sugar, blood pressure, cholesterol levels, and prevention of blood clots with aspirin will prevent complications.

Sadly, diabetes is generally not well controlled in the United States. Most diabetics have elevated average blood sugar levels. Blood pressure and cholesterol levels are not generally adequately controlled.

Why is this?

Patients are often blamed for not eating correctly and not losing weight. This is an easy excuse that in general is not true and based in many myths. One myth is that if a patient would eat a "healthy diet" there would be no problem. In fact, a "healthy diet" can be loaded with carbohydrates, and carbohydrates are precisely what diabetics cannot tolerate. Every diabetic's blood sugar will respond differently to a set carbohydrate load. The amount of carbohydrate an individual can tolerate can only be determined by measuring the blood sugar changes after meals.

Another myth is that if the patient would expend more effort to lose weight, the pounds would melt away. However, the truth is that as diet books fill library shelves and become a staple of the publishing industry, the number of obese and severely obese persons is increasing exponentially. Diabetes often needs to be controlled with complicated combinations of medications, meticulous attention to diet, exercise, and frequent blood sugar monitoring. To quote the character of Willy Loman in *Death of a Salesman* "attention must be paid." Diabetes has to be taken seriously!

Blood pressure and especially cholesterol levels should be significantly lower than those considered normal in nondiabetic individuals. Data from the Framingham study show that a diabetic with a cholesterol level of 180 has a greater risk of a heart attack than a nondiabetic patient with a cholesterol level of 360. A previously healthy diabetic has the same risk of a heart attack as someone who already has had a heart attack. Many physicians are not aware of the magnitude of a diabetic's increased cardiovascular risk.

Judith McQuown has had diabetes for eighteen years. As a patient she has to deal with the disease continuously. Physician interaction is usually brief, and practical advice is very limited. It is gratifying for me as a physician to see that Judith has taken charge of her own diabetes. Judith has done her own research and come to her own conclusions out of necessity. She has read widely and uncovered a plethora of useful facts about the disease. Judith has spoken with countless other diabetics both in person and via the Internet.

This combination of personal observation, literature research, and information exchange is the basis of *1,001 Tips for Living Well with Diabetes*. The book contains invaluable pearls gleaned over literally millennia of combined diabetic practice. Judith is an accomplished author whose books have sold over 500,000 copies. She has done a spectacular job of assembling her tips and expressing them in a terse and witty style that readers will appreciate. The exposition is clear and to the point. Readers will definitely benefit from Judith's insights. They will also be encouraged to embrace their own diabetic experience and discover their own truths about diabetes. *1,001 Tips for Living Well with Diabetes* encourages the attention that must be paid in order to control the disease.

A caveat must be stated. Every diabetic is different. Every tip is not applicable to every diabetic. Diabetic truths can often be personal and not universal. Readers should evaluate whether a particular tip is applicable to themselves and to consult their physicians for guidance.

—HARRY GRUENSPAN, MD, PHD
Assistant Attending Physician
Presbyterian Hospital / The New York Hospital
Cornell Medical Center
Instructor in Medicine
Cornell University

Introduction

THIS IS A book full of hope and practicality.

This is a book with hundreds of ideas you can use to live well despite your diabetes.

You probably know that diabetes is now classified as a pandemic (worldwide epidemic). It even rated a *Time* magazine cover story in December 2003.

The statistics are staggering. According to the World Health Organization, 177 million people had diabetes in 2000—33 million in India and 23 million in China—and 300 million people are projected to have diabetes in 2025.

Most of these people have type 2 diabetes, which is associated with obesity and inactivity. Obesity affects three times as many people in the United Kingdom as twenty years ago and could rise to 40 percent of the population by 2020. That could lead to the first drop in British life expectancy in over a century because obesity shortens people's lives. The more they weigh, the more likely they are to die young.

In the United States, there are over 18 million people with diabetes; more than 1.2 million new cases were diagnosed last year. Of these, 2.7 million are African-American, 2.0 million are Hispanic, 0.1 million are Native Americans living on reservations—but some tribes have a 50 percent diabetes rate—9.3 million are women, and 8.6 million are senior citizens. (Obviously, some people with diabetes belong to two or three of these categories.)

Countless millions more have started on the road to diabetes. Known variously as "metabolic syndrome" or "Syndrome X," this condition is defined by the National Institutes of Health as a person's having at least three out of five of the following symptoms:

- heavy abdominal fat, with a waistline over 40 inches for men, over 35 inches for women
- blood pressure higher than 130/85
- HDL (good) cholesterol lower than 40 mg./dl.
- triglycerides higher than 150 mg./dl.
- fasting blood sugar higher than 110 mg./dl.

At least 47 million American adults—more than 20 percent of the population—have metabolic syndrome, which affects more than 40 percent of Americans in their sixties and seventies.

"Prediabetes" is another condition that leads to full-blown diabetes if left unchecked. An estimated 41 million Americans have the condition, which is identified by a blood sugar level higher than 100 mg./dl.

The tips in this book are designed to help these people, too. With a little care, self-discipline, and good medical treatment, they will be able to avoid or postpone the onset of diabetes and to minimize its potential damage.

The annual economic cost of diabetes in 2002 has been estimated at $132 billion, or 10 percent of every health-care dollar spent in the United States. Many experts fear that diabetes' annual costs could bankrupt Social Security by 2025.

Ever wondered why? Let's look at some scary statistics:

- The average American eats more than 158 pounds of sugar per year.
- 25 percent of all vegetables eaten in the United States are French fries.
- American spending on fast food has risen 18 times (1700 percent) in the past thirty years.

As a result, today's American children may be the first modern generation to have shorter life expectancies than their parents.

Today's Battle of the Bulge is far more lethal than the one we fought and won sixty years ago. That World War II battle suffered more than 180,000 casualties in six weeks of fighting. This battle is ongoing and will result in millions of diabetes-related deaths throughout the world in the next decade alone. Both type 2s, who often battle overweight and obesity, and type 1s, who may not have weight problems, are at risk and must plan for their healthy futures.

Think of your diabetes as a time bomb with a very long fuse. It's a time bomb because eventually it could cause heart disease, stroke, kidney disease, blindness, and some forms of cancer.

But its long fuse means that you can take action to prevent or delay those deadly diseases and live a long, happy, productive life.

PERSONAL HISTORY: I was diagnosed as a type 2 diabetic in 1987, although I had probably been a diabetic for two or three years at that point. After a six-month "honeymoon" on oral hypoglycemics, I had to be switched to insulin. I have now been on insulin for seventeen years.

Thanks to the advances in diabetes research over the past seventeen years, I now know that it is probable that I had type 1.5 diabetes, also known as LADA (Latent Autoimmune Diabetes in Adults) or Slow Onset Type 1. I don't think that it makes much difference now. We can't change the past. But we can make changes now to improve our future health.

In the seventeen years that I have had diabetes, I have learned many things. The two most important have been: keep learning about this disease because there have been and will be so many advances in research and treatment, and always have a sense of humor and a "Plan B" so that life's little curves and uncertainties don't create stress.

The tips in these chapters come from many sources: friends and friends of friends all over the United States, parents and teachers of children with diabetes, doctors and researchers, a support group in New York City, and many people I met online. Many of these tips are my own, based on personal experience.

The tips in these chapters may seem to be random. That's because I want you to *read each one separately* and think about it for a minute. In that way, the tips will be of the greatest help to you and your family.

You will notice that nearly half the tips are concentrated in two chapters: "Weight Loss and Nutrition" and "Dealing with Depression and Stress." That is because I believe that if you lose weight, eat more healthily, and overcome depression and stress at least half the time, you will manage your diabetes successfully.

I have not included any tips about insulin pumps because these marvelous machines have already been covered exhaustively in Gabrielle Kaplan-Mayer's excellent book, *Insulin Pump Therapy Demystified* (Marlowe & Company, 2003).

Here's the most important tip:

1 **BE CREATIVE!** ■ Regard diabetes as a challenge that you can outsmart. Think "outside the box" to solve problems and achieve results.

It's up to you—these tips will help!

1

Drugs and Equipment

2   **NO DRUG WORKS FOR EVERYONE** ■ Every patient is a unique individual. Not only does no drug work for everyone, but it is very likely that, as time passes, your body will get used to a drug you are taking, or that your condition progresses (or both), and you will have to change the dosage of the drug or even switch to another drug.

Fortunately, there are many drugs for the treatment of diabetes—and even more in the pipeline—so your doctor's changing them shouldn't be a problem.

3   **MANY DRUGS TAKE GETTING USED TO** ■ When your doctor gives you a new or different drug, or a new dosage or formulation, it may take several days to a week for your body to get used to it and for it to work well.

If you have an adverse reaction, call your doctor immediately. Otherwise, give the drug a chance to work.

4   **WEIGHT LOSS CAN LOWER YOUR DRUG REQUIREMENTS** ■ Even if you have lost only ten or fifteen pounds, you may need to have your medication changed. Call your doctor, especially if you start having two or three low blood-glucose readings per week.

5 **TEST OFTEN** ■ If you use insulin, you should be testing your blood glucose at least three or four times a day. Most of us long-termers on insulin test more than five times a day. If you're not on insulin you might be tempted to test less frequently—some diabetics test once a day or less—but the more often you test, the more precise information you have about your blood glucose numbers, and the better you can take care of yourself.

Test-strip suppliers—usually connected with HMOs—will generally give you only five or six test strips a day—500 for a three-month period. But they don't always tell you that you can get more without having to buy them.

All you need is a doctor's prescription with the magic words "medical necessity," the number of times a day you test, and the total number of strips you need for the allotted time period. Doctors, HMOs, and insurance companies are usually happy to do this because they know that the more frequently you test, the less likely it is that you will develop expensive diabetic complications.

6 **MINIMIZE THE STICKING POINT** ■ If you test your blood glucose several times a day with a lancet, in time your fingertips and other parts of your anatomy will resemble a pincushion. Insulin users can minimize these holes by using the needle from their last insulin syringe, after wiping it with an alcohol swab to sterilize it. The needle is much thinner, so it inflicts less damage to your tissues—and less pain.

(However, my friend Mischa, who is much taller and outweighs me by 90 pounds, argues that a lancet has a major advantage for the squeamish. *It* does the work, rather than your having to do the finger sticks yourself.)

Choose the instrument and method that makes you feel the most comfortable. When insulin needles are thinner than lancets, you may prefer doing finger sticks with them. When newer, thinner lancets are available, you may want to switch—and use them with or without the lancing device.

7 **SYRINGE SMARTS** ■ As syringe needles have become progressively shorter and thinner, I have changed sizes three or four times in the past ten years. Thinner, shorter needles cause less tissue damage and are less painful. Pharmacists and manufacturers' Web sites as well as physicians are excellent sources of what's new.

8 **DOUBLE UP ON YOUR INSULIN** ■ Until Murphy's Law is repealed, the one time a year that you drop a bottle of insulin and break it is during a three-day blizzard.

Remember the Boy Scout motto. Being prepared prevents panic and emergencies.

Always make sure that you have at least two bottles of every type of insulin you are taking. As many insurance companies will pay for only *one* bottle at a time, ask your doctor to write "medical necessity" on the prescription so that your insurance company will let you have two bottles at one time without making you pay for the second one.

9 **FINESSING THE 72-HOUR TEST** ■ The 72-hour blood-glucose test is a useful tool for diagnosing when, how, and why some diabetics experience gyrating blood-glucose levels for no apparent reason, a condition known as "brittle diabetes."

A physician or nurse inserts a tiny sensor that takes minute blood samples every five minutes, into your abdomen and tapes it securely. These samples are transmitted to a monitor clipped onto your waistband or underwear (or pajamas when you're asleep). The monitor registers these 864 blood-glucose readings, which are downloaded into a computer and analyzed at the end of the 72 hours. During the test, ERROR messages and beeps will alert you to problems.

Unfortunately, this equipment can malfunction, and the test will have to be aborted. A company representative told me that this happens a little more than 10 percent of the time. (My estimate is closer to 20 percent after two of my tests in two months with different sensors and monitors had to be aborted.)

Undeterred, I decided to create a modified test. I urge you to try it, too, if your monitor malfunctions, or if your insurance does not cover the test. My endocrinologist found this detailed data very useful in fine-tuning my insulin dosages.

Choose a three-day weekend, or three consecutive days when you can work from home. Do finger sticks every hour on the hour (or as close to it as you can) from the time you wake up until bedtime and, if possible, at least once during the middle of the night. Keep a detailed log of your readings. Also log in your insulin dosages, other medication, meals, exercise, and hypoglycemic "events." Your goal is to have at least forty-five blood-glucose readings over three days. Admittedly, it's a lot of work, but it's only three days, and your doctor's analyzing the results will give you better control of your diabetes.

Some critics of this strategy feel that doing the test during three consecutive days in the workplace/office produces more accurate results. However, other medical professionals believe that testing your blood glucose every hour on the hour while working in your office could create so much stress that the blood-glucose numbers would be high and therefore inaccurate. It's a very individual decision, but I'll vote with the second group.

10 **IF YOUR INSURANCE DOESN'T COVER TESTING SUPPLIES ■** Many experienced diabetics use eBay to purchase testing supplies and recommend it to others. They urge bidding at the last moment so they cannot be outbid.

Make sure you check information on expiration dates, shipping costs, payment methods, and customer feedback on the seller. E-mail the seller if detailed shipping information is not provided, or if you have any questions.

11 **WHEN HALF MEASURES WORK BEST ■** Although this tip seems obvious, few doctors suggest it. Often—especially in newly diagnosed Type I (insulin-dependent) diabetics—10 (or any whole number of units of insulin) is too little, but 11 is too much.

Syringes are designed with enough space between units to get midpoints, so you can measure 10½ units pretty accurately. With your doctor's approval, try this dosage for at least three days and see if your results improve.

12 **WHEN PILLS WORK TOO QUICKLY** ■ Similarly, in some diabetics, oral hypoglycemics kick in too quickly, causing rapid drops in blood glucose. For a slower, smoother evening out, ask your doctor whether a time-release oral hypoglycemic would work better for you.

13 **POST-9/11 TRAVEL RULES** ■ Official Policy: Increased security since September 11, 2001 means that you will have to prove that your syringes, insulin, blood-glucose meter, test strips, glucagon, and other gear are for your diabetes and that it is medically necessary for you to carry them. If you are wearing a pump, you will have to show that to airport security, too.

Now you will need a recent letter from your doctor stating that you are a diabetic and that you need to carry all these drugs and equipment. Most important, you will need to carry your insulin in the prescription box it came in, and at least one *unopened* package of syringes as well as the syringes you need, so that airport security can verify your loose syringes are identical to the packaged ones.

Although this is the official policy, it does not appear to be enforced consistently or as strongly as these paragraphs suggest. Many travelers with diabetes have never had their drugs or diabetes supplies questioned and have never been asked to produce a letter from their doctor.

14 **LANTUS: THE "POOR PATIENT'S PUMP"** ■ Lantus, the newest long-acting insulin, is a godsend for many diabetics whose blood glucose yo-yo'd on Ultralente and other long-acting insulins. Because Lantus has a duration of approximately 24 hours, it provides a basal level that mimics the action of a normal pancreas, or of a pump that releases small doses of insulin continually.

With Lantus, you will still have to use a fast-acting insulin like Humalog or Novolog to cover meals, and you will have to use *separate* syringes for Lantus and the fast-acting insulin because they react with each other. However, if Lantus gives you better blood-glucose control, you may be able to skip your before-lunch or before-dinner Humalog.

15 **"MY DIABETES ISN'T SERIOUS BECAUSE I'M ONLY TAKING PILLS" IS A DANGEROUS MYTH** ■ Many type 2 diabetics don't take their disease seriously enough. They say, "My diabetes isn't serious because I don't have to take insulin. I'm only taking pills."

And then, because it isn't "serious," they act as if they don't have diabetes at all: They don't test their blood glucose and they don't watch their carbohydrate intake. Many type 2s are overweight or even clinically obese, but make no attempt to diet.

Over the years, this cavalier behavior causes serious, irreversible damage, like neuropathy, retina problems, and gangrene. One of my type 2 "non-insulin-dependent" friends who disregarded diet and exercise for years is waiting for a kidney transplant and may have to go on dialysis before then. Both are unpleasant options.

How you take care of yourself *now* is an investment in your healthy *future*.

16 **STARTING INSULIN THERAPY IMMEDIATELY MAY BE A SMART MOVE** ■ You are a newly diagnosed type 2 diabetic, which means that your pancreas is making insulin. But your doctor recommends insulin injections anyway. How come?

Recent research suggests that many new type 2s are stressing their pancreases in the early days of their disease. That's why there is often a "honeymoon" of several months to a year when oral medications work, followed by an inevitable burnout, when their pancreases stop manufacturing insulin. At that point, they must take insulin for the rest of their lives.

However, if you are put on insulin immediately, your overburdened pancreas is able to rest and recuperate. Later—especially if you are able to go from obesity to overweight, or overweight to normal weight—you may be able to switch from insulin to pills.

17

TIMING YOUR LANTUS CAN MAKE A BIG DIFFERENCE ▪ Taking your Lantus (very long-acting insulin) in the morning rather than before bedtime seems to work better. A recent study of 695 adult-onset diabetics who were taking insulin *and* oral medication to better control their blood glucose found that the patients who took Lantus in the early morning controlled their blood glucose better than those who took it at bedtime, and both groups did better than patients who took NPH, a different type of insulin, at bedtime.

Although researchers couldn't explain why the morning injection of Lantus gave the best results, it's certainly worth discussing changing the timing with your doctor.

18

DOUBLE-CHECK IF YOUR TEST RESULTS LOOK STRANGE ▪ Every so often, you'll get a blood-glucose result that looks strange. It's way too high or too low, but you don't feel any different.

Before adjusting your medication or popping a glucose tablet, double-check. First, make sure that the area you're taking blood from is absolutely clean. Fingertips especially can pick up trace amounts of food or other substances that can distort your test results.

Then make sure that the sample is really all blood—not half blood and half clear fluid, which can happen in cold weather. See that it fills the test chamber completely.

If this test result is substantially different from the first, repeat the test a third time. The second and third tests should show similar readings. Use an average of these two readings to get a fairly accurate test result.

19

A GLUCAGON KIT CAN SAVE YOUR LIFE ▪ If you have ever fainted from severe hypoglycemia (or come close), you must keep a glucagon kit handy for future emergencies when you are unable to swallow.

Glucagon is a hormone that raises your blood sugar by increasing the rate at which glycogen, which is stored in the liver, breaks down and is converted into glucose. It works very quickly.

As preparing and injecting the glucagon is a little complex, have one or more family members or close friends familiarize themselves with the location of the kit and the instructions. They should also practice by giving you your insulin shot now and then.

It is imperative that your designated "medic" act quickly. The longer you are unconscious, the more dangerous it is. Brain damage can start in thirty minutes!

Unfortunately, glucagon kits are useless if you live alone. When your blood glucose drops to 30 or 40, you are too uncoordinated to mix the glucagon and to inject it. If you even *suspect* that your blood glucose is tanking, jam some glucose tablets into your mouth and chew and swallow them quickly.

Note: Sometimes two injections are needed, so you may want to keep two kits on hand. Fortunately, they can be kept at room temperature, and they have a shelf life of over one year.

20 **PARTICIPATE IN A CLINICAL TRIAL** ■ Most clinical trials for promising new drugs are for Phase II (efficacy), Phase III (the new drug vs. drugs already in use or vs. a standard treatment), or a combined Phase II/III study.

These drugs have already passed Phase I (safety) trials and been approved by the Food & Drug Administration for further study.

When you volunteer for a clinical trial, there is a possibility that you will receive the placebo rather than the new drug. In fact, in double-blind studies, which are the most common type, the experimenters do not know which patients are getting the new drug and which the placebo.

In either case, however, you should receive superb medical care from some of the most talented and attentive doctors and researchers in the United States. And you may help with the discovery of a miraculous new drug!

21 **REPLACE YOUR INSULIN FREQUENTLY** ■ Remember these guidelines to keep your insulin potent:

▶ An unopened vial stored in the refrigerator should last until the expiration date. However, just to make sure, start using it at least two months before the expiration date.

▶ An unopened vial stored at room temperature lasts 28 days.

▶ An opened vial stored in the refrigerator lasts 28 days.

▶ An opened vial stored at room temperature lasts 28 days.

22 **CHOOSE SUGAR-FREE MEDICATIONS** ■ Many over-the-counter medications, like cough syrups and antacids, contain sugar, which creates a problem in controlling your blood glucose.

Read labels carefully. Choose drugs that display "sugar-free" wording prominently. Ask your doctor or pharmacist for advice.

23 **THE STATIN SOLUTION** ■ Cholesterol-lowering statin drugs like Lescol (fluvastatin), Mevacor (lovastatin), Pravachol (pravastatin) and Zocor (simvastatin) are being prescribed for people with diabetes even if their cholesterol is low or normal. Using these drugs daily can cut the risk of heart disease and stroke in diabetics by about one-third.

Note: If you take statins, tell your doctor if you experience muscle aches and pains, which are fairly common side effects. Also, make sure that your liver enzymes are checked every three months. Elevated liver enzymes can be reversed by altering the type of statin or lowering the dosage of the drug.

24 **GAUGE SIZE MAKES A BIG DIFFERENCE** ■ Needle and lancet sizes are stated in wire gauge, whose numbers look pretty close together: 28, 30, 31, 33 gauge. But there is a great difference.

GAUGE SIZE	MILLIMETERS
28	0.32
30	0.25
31	0.22
33	0.18

Note that as the gauge increases, the size in millimeters decreases.

A little quick arithmetic shows you that a 33-gauge lancet is 28 percent smaller than a 30-gauge lancet, and a 31-gauge syringe needle is 12 percent smaller than a 30-gauge syringe needle. Your fingers and other test sites and insulin injection sites will definitely notice the difference: less pain and less tissue damage.

25 **AVOID PRESCRIPTION ERRORS ■** A recent survey found that *half* the pharmacists interviewed admitted that they had filled a prescription incorrectly because of the doctor's sloppy handwriting. That explains why drug error is the cause of 140,000 deaths per year.

To avoid errors in your prescriptions, ask your doctor to spell out the name of the medication and write it down, along with the correct dosage and time(s) you should take it. When you pick up the prescription, compare the label with your notes.

You can minimize the chance of errors even more by getting your prescription filled in the early afternoon, the slowest time of the day, when pharmacist mistakes are the least likely.

26 **PILL SPLITTERS CUT YOUR DRUG BILLS IN HALF ■** This strategy works best (a) when your drug plan has a flat copayment per drug per month regardless of the dosage; (b) your medication is a pill that comes in several dosages; (c) your doctor is willing to write a prescription for pills that are double your dosage and tells you that it is OK for you to split these pills in half.

Buy a pill splitter at your pharmacy—it should cost around $3–$5. Then follow the directions to cut a pill in half, take half (this is your regular dosage), and wrap the other half in plastic for your next dose. Doing this will turn one month's supply into two, thus cutting your drug bill in half.

27 **KEEP ANTIBIOTICS HANDY ■** Do you catch the same kind of "bug" every year? Like a strep throat? Does your doctor prescribe the same antibiotic? Then it's a good idea to start taking that antibiotic quickly to prevent a long, serious illness that might lead to hospitalization. One savvy diabetic and her doctor agreed on this game plan so that she can start treatment immediately.

Her doctor gave her a prescription for ten days' worth of an antibiotic that she has taken successfully for many years, and she filled it and put it away.

When she becomes sick, she tries aspirin, vitamin C, and chicken soup for two or three days. Then she calls her doctor to make sure her symptoms sound like those of a bacterial infection. If her doctor gives her the OK, she starts the antibiotic without risking exposure to other "bugs" in his waiting room.

But if she is still sick after two or three days on the antibiotic, she *must* call her doctor and come in for an examination and lab tests.

This treatment strategy has worked so well that she has fought the bug and avoided serious complications for many years—all by having her antibiotics within arm's reach.

28 FLEXIBLE INSULIN ■ In a perfect world, we would start eating a meal between thirty and forty-five minutes after injecting insulin.

But in the real world, we might inject insulin, go to a restaurant or dinner party, order, and then wait and wait as our blood glucose drops, knowing that the insulin and our food will not coincide.

However, Humalog is a faster-acting, more flexible insulin. Not only can it be injected *just before* you eat, it can also be taken *immediately after* you eat. In fact, you might even think of Humalog as an "oops!" or "morning-after" drug because if you overeat at dinner or a party, you can adjust your dosage immediately afterward to compensate for the extra carbohydrates.

29 DON'T BLAME YOURSELF IF YOU NEED TO INCREASE YOUR DOSAGE ■ After being on a medication for some time, the human body often stops responding to it as effectively. We need more of it—or maybe even a new or different drug—to achieve the desired result.

Don't blame yourself. It happens all the time—just ask any doctor or pharmacist.

30 HOW LONG WILL IT TAKE? ■ When your doctor prescribes a new drug, ask how long it will take for you to see results. This is *almost* as important as asking about side effects.

31 UPDATE YOUR IMMUNIZATIONS ■ You need diphtheria and tetanus booster shots every ten years. If you don't remember the last time you had a booster shot, it's probably time to get one. For more information, contact Immunization Action Coalition, (651) 647-9009 or log on to www.immunize.org.

32 ALWAYS ASK FOR GENERIC DRUGS ■ Many generic versions of prescription drugs are available, and they can save you big bucks. The average cost of a generic drug is $14, compared with $77 for the average brand-name prescription.

The Food and Drug Administration (FDA) requires generics to be identical to the original brand-name drugs in dosage, quality, safety, and strength, although their appearance and inactive ingredients may differ.

33 MULTIVITAMIN BENEFITS FOR TYPE 2S ■ A daily multivitamin/mineral may reduce infections in people with type 2 diabetes. In a study reported in *Annals of Internal Medicine*, one group of type 2 diabetics took a daily multivitamin; the control group took a placebo (inert pill). After a year, only 17 percent of the vitamin group reported an infectious illness, compared with 93 percent who took the placebo. And the vitamin group reported *no* illness-related work absences, compared to 89 percent taking the placebo who reported at least one absence.

34 COFFEE REDUCES DIABETES RISK ■ Actually, it's the caffeine in coffee that makes it so beneficial. As caffeine is often treated as a drug, I've put the tip in this chapter.

Harvard Public Health researchers followed 42,888 men and 85,056 women from 1980 to 1998. According to the standards of the time, none of them had diabetes at the beginning of the study. Men who drank more than six cups of caffeinated coffee per day cut their risk of type 2 diabetes by about 50 percent. Women who drank that much coffee cut their risk by 30 percent. The Harvard researchers believe that the caffeine affects the way the body metabolizes sugar, thus lowering the risk of type 2 diabetes.

Note: There was a more modest effect among decaf drinkers (25 percent risk reduction for men and 15 percent for women) and no statistically significant connection between type 2 diabetes risk and tea, which also contains caffeine.

35 CONGESTIVE HEART FAILURE? DON'T TAKE THESE DIABETES DRUGS ■ The Food and Drug Administration has warned explicitly that metformin (Glucophage) and thiazolidinediones (TZDs) like Avandia and Actos should not be taken by patients with congestive heart failure as well as diabetes.

Unfortunately, as the use of these diabetes drugs has been rising over the past six years, one study showed that a significant percentage of hospital Medicare recipients with both diseases were discharged with a metformin or TZD prescription.

If you suffer from both congestive heart failure and diabetes, ask your doctor for diabetes drugs that do not impact congestive heart failure.

36 THE PEN: MIGHTIER THAN THE SYRINGE? ■ Well, insulin pens—both prefilled disposable pens and insulin cartridges in reusable pens—are more convenient than syringes. And the pens are very accurate, especially for low doses of insulin.

One of the problems with greater U.S. adoption of insulin pens is that the Food and Drug Administration considers prefilled disposable pens to be drugs because they are self-contained. As such they are often reimbursed by insurance companies. In contrast, reusable pens are generally not reimbursed, although the insulin cartridges are.

However, this is an area that is still evolving. In Europe, most insulin-dependent diabetics already use insulin pens, which are covered by the country's health-care system.

37 **LANCING DEVICES: THERE *IS* A CHOICE ■** Many insulin-dependent diabetics don't mind taking their insulin injections, but they hate checking their blood sugars. And the great majority of type 2 diabetics really hate the procedure because the lancing device is hard to use or penetrates too deeply and painfully.

Remembering that you will test your blood sugars many thousands of times in your lifetime, it's definitely worth considering using lancets without the device and its scary, uncomfortable trigger, or finding a device with a dial-a-depth feature, so that you can use different depth settings for different fingers.

38 **DO THE PILL DRILL ■** Get a pill container marked with the days of the week with seven to twenty-one compartments, depending on your needs. Fill it once a week, then use it every day.

This strategy has two advantages. First, you save time by doing this job once, rather than every day. Second, you know immediately whether you have taken your medications, rather than the occasional "Did I or didn't I?"

39 **GIVE YOUR FINGERTIPS A REST ■** Unless you are checking for hypoglycemia, when only your fingertips will give you an accurate result, use other test sites and give your fingertips a rest.

Try your forearm, upper arm, calf, thigh, or the palm of your hand several inches below your thumb or your pinkie, close to your wrist. These areas have fewer nerve endings, so testing there will usually be less painful.

40 TAKE YOUR PILLS PROPERLY ■ Get the full benefit from your medications by understanding what the instructions mean.

"Before meals"—at least one hour before eating

"After meals"—at least two hours after eating

"With food"—during or just after a meal, not with just a glass of juice or milk

"On an empty stomach"—one hour before or two hours after eating

41 BE WARY OF ONLINE PHARMACIES ■ Ordering over the Internet can be tempting, and millions of people do, to the tune of an estimated $15 billion in 2004. While many e-pharmacies are legitimate and require a faxed or mailed prescription from a licensed doctor who has given you a physical exam, many others are not. They will supply drugs without prescriptions. Sometimes people can get them by listing fake symptoms on the sites' medical questionnaires.

Online drugs may not be such a bargain. Many e-pharmacies inflate their "bargain" prices with enormous consultation and shipping fees. And some sites can steal your money and personal identity.

To protect yourself, use only sites authorized by the Verified Internet Pharmacy Practice Sites program. Make sure the sites are secure, so that your credit-card information can't be stolen, and never give out your Social Security number or passwords.

The bottom line? Buyer beware.

42 TRANSLATE YOUR GLYCOSYLATED HEMOGLOBIN A1C NUMBERS ■ It may be difficult to relate the single-digit hemoglobin A1C percentages to two- and three-digit blood-glucose figures. This table does the translation for you:

A1C	AVERAGE BLOOD GLUCOSE
5%	100
6	135
7	170

A1C	AVERAGE BLOOD GLUCOSE
8	205
9	240
10	275
11	310
12	345
13	380

As you can see, each whole percent is equivalent to 35 points of blood glucose, so 0.1 percent equals 3.5 points.

That said, a difference of even 0.2–0.5 between two tests is not serious and is not statistically significant. A difference of a whole percentage point is.

43 REALIZE THAT THE GLYCOSYLATED HEMOGLOBIN A1C TEST IS AN AVERAGE ■ Remember that this test is an arithmetic average. Like the story of the man who drowned in a pond whose average depth was only 18 inches, it's possible to have a "good" reading of 6% (135 blood glucose) that is really an average of much higher and much lower blood-glucose numbers.

44 DON'T REUSE LANCETS ■ Well, if you absolutely must, make sure that you've sterilized them by soaking them in alcohol. Reusing lancets to check your blood glucose raises the risk of dangerous finger infections. In rare cases, when lancets are used many times, these infections can become persistent and very difficult to cure.

45 BETTER BLOOD-GLUCOSE CONTROL CAN MEAN LESS MEDICATION ■ Sometimes better control—achieving lower blood-sugar numbers—can mean reducing the dosage of your oral hypoglycemic drugs. Some of my friends have cut their metformin dosage in half: from 1,000 mg. twice a day to 1,000 mg. after breakfast.

And sometimes better control can mean cutting down on insulin or, in the case of people with type 2 diabetes, getting off insulin completely and using oral medication alone.

46 DON'T GET PRESCRIPTIONS FILLED ON SUNDAY ■ This may sound like the old slogan, "Don't buy a car built on Monday"—and it is.

Pharmacists who fill in on Sundays are usually not familiar with all the drugs that all their customers are taking. They don't know enough to question when something looks wrong, whether it's the prescription itself or just the insurance copayment. When was I charged the full retail price for a prescription—and didn't realize it until I got home because I was given a thirty-day supply instead of the usual ninety-day supply? On Sunday, of course. That's how and why I wrote this tip.

47 NOTE THE BIG DIFFERENCE BETWEEN 70/30 INSULIN AND 75/25 INSULIN ■ It looks like just a 5 percent differential, but it's a big difference that may make mealtimes easier for you.

Both are premixed insulins. However, the 70/30 mixture should be taken 30–45 minutes before eating. The Humalog Mix 75/25 is taken within 15 minutes before eating, which can give you greater flexibility.

48 TWO SEPARATE INSULINS MAY WORK BETTER FOR YOU ■ However, some diabetics who use insulin get better control from being able to calibrate specific doses of both their long- and short-acting insulins, rather than being locked into just increasing or decreasing the number of units of a fixed blend.

It can take several months for you and your doctor to figure out which system is better for you. Keeping a careful diary of blood-glucose readings, diet, and exercise is crucial.

49 YOUR INSULIN SHOULDN'T BE ICE-COLD ■ If you keep your insulin in the refrigerator and injecting it hurts, take your vial(s) out thirty minutes before you inject it so that the insulin will be at room temperature. That will make it less painful.

50 **ROTATE YOUR INJECTION SITES** ■ You can always use the same, least painful area of your body so long as you rotate your injection sites. For example, you can always inject insulin into your abdomen—avoiding your navel—if you rotate the exact location.

One easy method is to picture your abdomen as a clock and place each injection at the next hour marking. When you have circled the clock on your left side, switch to the right. That will give you plenty of time to heal and avoid internal scarring, which can affect the proper absorption of the insulin.

51 **SOME INSULINS CAN BE INJECTED ANYWHERE, SOME CAN'T** ■ Slower-acting insulins like Lantus, Ultralente, Lente, and Regular can be injected anywhere in the body where there is enough fat to avoid injecting into the muscle. But Humalog—the fastest-acting insulin—should be injected only into the abdomen, so that it is absorbed most rapidly.

52 **CHECK YOUR PRESCRIPTIONS BEFORE YOU LEAVE THE PHARMACY** ■ Go one step further than just checking the label. Open the bottle and examine the pills themselves. If a pill looks different from what you're used to, check that the code printed on the pill is identical to the code printed on the label. (The Web site www.rxlist.com lets you type in the code and get the name and the dosage of the drug, or ask the pharmacist to do it for you.)

Note: Sometimes a pharmacy may substitute twice as many pills that are half your usual dosage if it runs out of your prescribed dose, but your pharmacist should instruct you to take twice as many of the pills.

53 USE A NATIONAL PHARMACY CHAIN ■ You're in a faraway city when suddenly you realize you forgot to pack your medication. But that's no problem if you use a national pharmacy chain. Just ask the pharmacist in the city you're visiting to check your prescription online, explain that you need a week's refill of your medications, and you'll be able to get them.

54 HAVE YOUR PHARMACY'S FAX NUMBER HANDY ■ Sometimes your doctor can't get through on the phone, or it's not convenient to call the pharmacy immediately. Being able to give your pharmacy's fax number to your doctor—or being able to use it yourself—gives you another way to get your prescriptions filled.

55 GET FAMILIAR WITH THE FORMULARY ■ Most health-insurance plans have a formulary: a list of brand-name and generic drugs for which they will pay, and leave you with the usually reasonable copay.

But if your doctor prescribes a drug that is not in the formulary, *you* will have to pay the full retail price, and it can be horrendous. For example, Cipro antibiotic ear drops, which were not in my medical group's formulary, cost $110; Cortisporin, a similar brand-name antibiotic ear drop, cost only $10 for the copay.

To save yourself time and aggravation, when your doctor gives you a new prescription, ask whether the drug is in the formulary. If your doctor doesn't know, ask whether the prescription can be written so that an equivalent formulary-acceptable brand-name or generic drug can be substituted.

56 IMPAIRED GLUCOSE TOLERANCE (IGT) AND IMPAIRED FASTING GLUCOSE (IFG) MAY REQUIRE DIFFERENT DRUGS ■ According to a recent six-year British study, people with impaired glucose tolerance (IGT) and impaired fasting glucose (IFG) may need different treatment to prevent type 2 diabetes.

People who had IGT and took Precose (acarbose) significantly reduced their risk of developing type 2 diabetes, compared to the people in the study who took metformin, the generic form of Glucophage. But among the people with IFG, there was no significant difference in the risk of developing diabetes between those who took Precose and those who took metformin.

The difference in the IGT results may be due to the difference in the ways the two drugs work: Precose delays carbohydrate absorption, which reduces rises in blood glucose after eating. Metformin restricts the liver's ability to release glucose into the blood.

57 MOVING TO INSULIN DOESN'T MEAN YOU'VE FAILED ■ Over time, many people with type 2 diabetes will progress from taking oral medications to needing to take insulin. This does not signify failure, and it doesn't necessarily mean that you're getting worse! It can simply mean that your pancreas is now producing less insulin, so supplementing your body's own supply is now necessary. Your doctor can refer you to a diabetes educator who will teach you how to inject and store insulin.

58 START INSULIN, GAIN WEIGHT? ■ Many people with type 2 diabetes who are put on insulin for better blood-glucose control discover that their weight skyrockets twenty to fifty pounds within one year. If this has been your experience, here's why it happened, and here's how to solve the problem:

Before you started on insulin, your body was not able to process carbohydrates efficiently, so the glucose that was produced was excreted in your urine, rather than going into your cells to be used. But on insulin, your body is able to use all those carbohydrates, so the result is a dramatic weight gain.

With all these calories and carbohydrates being used now, you won't feel as hungry or eat as much, but these changes take time. You should be able to lose your "insulin pounds" in about six months, but if you don't *start* losing weight within two weeks of starting on insulin, your dosage may need to be increased. (This may sound perplexing at first, but remember: *increased* insulin makes you *less* hungry.)

59 **VITAMIN E MAY REDUCE THE RISK OF TYPE 2 DIABETES** ■ A long-term Finnish study (1967–1995) reported in the February 27, 2004 issue of *Diabetes Care* concluded that there was a significant correlation between diets highest in vitamin E and a reduced risk of type 2 diabetes.

Vitamin E is also essential for cardiovascular health. It acts as a blood thinner, which reduces the risk of clots and helps keep LDL (bad) cholesterol from forming plaques that stick to artery walls and may cause blockages.

Note: Curiously, there was no statistical correlation between vitamin C and reduced risk of type 2 diabetes.

60 **DIURETICS CAN RAISE YOUR BLOOD GLUCOSE** ■ This tip may sound like the computer error message: "It's not my fault . . ." But if you have just been put on a diuretic (water pill) to lower your blood pressure, the concentration of glucose in your blood will probably rise.

If your high blood glucose lasts for more than two or three days while your body gets used to the diuretic, call your doctor. You may need to increase your insulin or oral hypoglycemic dosage, or use a lower dosage of the diuretic, or a different one.

61 **GET YOUR PHARMACY'S PACKAGE INSERT** ■ This long strip of paper with its tiny print and biochemical vocabulary is definitely worth reading and studying, even if you have to research the definitions of many technical words. Fortunately, the most important information is printed in bold type in clear English, e.g., "WARNINGS: Diabetes and Hypoglycemia . . ."

Besides pill splitting **(Tip No. 26)** and asking your doctor to prescribe generic drugs **(Tip No. 32)** there are other ways to pay less for your medications:

62 PAY LESS FOR PRESCRIPTION DRUGS I: ASK YOUR DOCTOR FOR SAMPLES ■ Doctors always have lots of sample drugs to give out to their patients. But if you don't say, "Do you have any samples of this?" you won't get any freebies.

Your simple request can save you big bucks. One man saved more than $350 last year because he asked his doctor for samples of Vioxx, a commonly prescribed arthritis drug. You may be able to get six months' worth of free samples in a single visit.

63 PAY LESS FOR PRESCRIPTION DRUGS II: IF THERE'S NO GENERIC ■ Some drugs are still under patent, so no generics are available. To find out if there is a generic equivalent, check the Food and Drug Administration's *Electronic Orange Book* (officially titled *Approved Drug Products with Therapeutic Equivalence Evaluations*) online at www.fda.gov/cder/ob/default.htm.

If your prescription is not available as a generic, ask your doctor if there is a *similar,* less expensive drug that can be prescribed instead.

64 PAY LESS FOR PRESCRIPTION DRUGS III: BUY THROUGH MAIL ORDER ■ The mail-order pharmacies discussed here are completely different from the online pharmacies I warned about earlier in this chapter **(Tip No. 41)**. These mail-order pharmacies have real addresses and phone numbers, and some of them are divisions of companies listed on the stock exchanges.

One simple way to find a reliable mail-order pharmacy is to ask your doctor or someone you trust for recommendations. Another is to look carefully at the pharmacy's Web site to check whether it requires a prescription and other information from your doctor, and whether it displays prominently the logo showing that it is a secure Web site.

These mail-order pharmacies can save their customers money because they may be located in low-rent or low-tax areas. Comparison-shop carefully. And these mail-order pharmacies may be worth using just because they are so convenient; most guarantee delivery in less than five days.

65 **PAY LESS FOR PRESCRIPTION DRUGS IV: BUY YOUR DRUGS IN BULK** ■ This strategy works especially well if you are taking prescription drugs for chronic or long-term problems. Unless doctors think you might misuse a drug, they are usually willing to write prescriptions for larger quantities, and pharmacies will fill those economy-size prescriptions.

How much can you save? One national pharmacy chain charges $10.99 for a one-month supply (30 100 mg. tablets) of Atenolol, a commonly prescribed hypertension drug. But a one-year supply (360 tablets) of the same drug cost only $54.49. The savings were $77.39—more than the cost of the one-year prescription!

For more expensive drugs, the savings are more amazing. Someone taking two Vioxx tablets a day for chronic arthritis pain was paying $242 for 100 tablets. But buying 300 at one time cost him only $369. His savings in one year were $869—almost two and one-half times the cost of his large-size prescription.

66 **PAY LESS FOR PRESCRIPTION DRUGS V: YOUR PHARMACIST MAY BE ABLE TO SUBSTITUTE** ■ Even if your doctor hasn't indicated that a generic drug can be substituted, ask your pharmacist about making the substitution. In most states, unless a prescription is marked specifically "Dispense as written," pharmacists are permitted to substitute the generic version of the proprietary (brand-name) drug.

67 **PAY LESS FOR PRESCRIPTION DRUGS VI: THE MOST IMPORTANT QUESTION TO ASK** ■ Many people with diabetes will be taking the same prescription drugs for the rest of their lives. Nevertheless, always ask your doctor, especially on repeat visits or when you are getting refill prescriptions, "Is it still necessary for me to take this drug?" It may not be—or something newer and better may have come along since your last visit.

2

Weight Loss and Nutrition

No Diet Is Right for Everyone

AS LONG-TERM dieters know, there is no "one-size-fits-all" diet. What works for you may not work for me, and vice versa. Although we both have diabetes, our body chemistry may be different, with one of us being able to metabolize carbohydrates fairly easily, with the help of oral hypoglycemics or insulin, and the other having trouble metabolizing those same carbohydrates, despite the help of oral hypoglycemics or insulin.

It may sound simplistic to say, "Do what works for you," but most of us have lived long enough to know whether we flourish under a high-carbohydrate or low-carbohydrate diet. Which diet helps us lose weight? Which one gives us more energy? Which one gives us better blood-glucose readings?

Many of the tips in this chapter have a low-carbohydrate bias because their contributors benefited from a low-carbohydrate diet and, probably, because they were disgruntled about being told constantly to go on a high-carbohydrate diet when empirically it made no sense to them. They had not succeeded with high-carbohydrate diets.

If I had to choose, I would stay away from the extremes of high- and low-carbohydrate diets. Probably neither 300 grams nor 30 grams of carbohydrate a day is healthy. A middle ground seems more sensible to me, more "Mediterranean" than Atkins Induction. Of course, the carbohydrates we choose should be complex, rather than simple and too quickly digested.

But that's just my humble opinion, and what's worked for me. Whatever diet you choose, have it checked by your doctor or Certified Diabetes Educator.

68 STAY AWAY FROM YOUR "TRIGGER" FOODS ■ We all have a love-hate relationship with certain foods: the ones that sing their siren song to us until we open the package—and then consume its entire contents. And then feel guilty as all get-out.

Very often, measuring out small portions of those beloved trigger foods doesn't work. We go back again and again and again.

The only effective strategy is to stay away from those foods completely—or to find a safer substitute, like air-popped popcorn instead of potato chips.

69 BETTER THAN BREADING ■ Most ingredients used to bread meat or fish for sautéing contain large percentages of carbohydrates: white or whole wheat flour, even nutritious wheat germ.

Finely chopped almonds are a better breading choice. The nuts contain protein, minerals, a little fat, and only a trace of carbohydrate. And they add lots of flavor and texture to your recipe. Big carb savings; one-quarter cup of all-purpose flour contains 24 grams of carbohydrate, one-quarter cup of chopped almonds, only 6 grams.

70 CREATE BEAUTY WITH ORIGAMI ■ I've put this tip into the Weight Loss and Nutrition chapter for a sneaky reason: Making origami prevents you from snacking for hours at a time.

Folding those beautiful papers so intricately and following complex instructions requires concentration. It's impractical to stop in the middle to grab a cookie, chip, or pretzel, then have to wash your hands and try to find your place again before continuing to create your origami pretties.

71 START WITH SOUP ■ Hot or cold, soup is an excellent starter. As you sip or spoon it, your brain and stomach begin to feel full. Consequently, you are likely to eat less of your main course and will take in fewer total calories. In fact, many successful diet plans are based on soup.

Here are some suggestions for quick, easy soups:

Cold: For all of these, you will need a blender and 1–2 cups of lowfat buttermilk per portion. Put the buttermilk in the blender. For Scandinavian-style fruit soups, add ½–1 cup of cut-up fresh apricots, cherries, raspberries, strawberries, or blueberries, As an extra treat, add 1 teaspoon rum, cognac, amaretto, or almond extract. Blend; chill; serve.

For cream of spinach, start with 1–2 cups of lowfat buttermilk per portion and put in blender. Thaw one-half of a 10-ounce package of frozen spinach, press out the water, and place in blender. Blend; chill; serve. Marvelous with grated nutmeg sprinkled on top.

Hot: Choose a low-sodium beef or chicken consommé. Some bouillon cubes are excellent. Top with chopped fresh or freeze-dried parsley.

72 SOUP CAN MAKE A MEAL ■ Take all the advantages in the preceding tip—and multiply them.

When you make soup your dinner, you are filling up on lots of low-calorie fluid. Here are some quick dinners based on revved-up soups:

Heat a can of chicken broth. Add a well-drained can of chicken breast and/or two beaten eggs, swirled with a fork through the soup. This is "egg drop" (without the high-carb cornstarch of the Cantonese version) or what Italian cooks call *stracciatella.* Top with fresh or freeze-dried chives.

Prepare a can of crabmeat soup according to the instructions. Add a well-drained 6-ounce can of crabmeat. For an extra treat, add 1 teaspoon cognac; the alcohol and calories will evaporate. Heat thoroughly and serve.

73 **GUILT-FREE POTATO CHIPS** ■ When you have an overpowering urge for potato chips, make your own to cut calories, carbohydrates, and fat. Store-bought chips are high in all three, so these snacks can really wreck your diet. For example, one company's potato chips contain 150 calories, 10 grams of fat, and 15 grams of carbohydrate in a 1-ounce serving. The company's baked variety contains 110 calories and only 1.5 grams of fat, but a whopping 23 grams of carbohydrate in a 1-ounce serving.

This recipe has only one disadvantage: You have to start the simple preparation the night before or the morning of your splurge.

Fill a 2- or 3-quart bowl with cold water. Scrub one or two potatoes; leave them unpeeled for extra minerals and flavor. Cut into thin slices, put into bowl of water, and refrigerate at least 8 hours. Then remove the potato slices with a slotted spoon or spatula and place on a paper towel.

You will notice that the bowl of water has a lot of white powder at the bottom. This is potato starch, which has been leached out of the potato slices, and is the source of most of the calories and carbohydrates.

Preheat your oven to 400 degrees. Spray a cookie sheet with vegetable spray—use butter or olive-oil flavor for extra taste. Place potato slices on the cookie sheet in a single layer. Bake 8–10 minutes per side, until golden brown. Serve.

I'd love to be able to give you a calorie and carbohydrate count for this recipe, but there are too many variables. The thinner you slice the potatoes and the longer they sit in the ice water, the more starch will be removed, and the lower the calorie and carbohydrate count will be. (The calories and fat grams in the cooking spray are negligible.) My estimate is that this recipe has only 30–40 calories and 5 grams of carbohydrate per 1-ounce serving.

74 **THE JOY OF JELL-O** ■ Sugar-free, that is. It's a perfect bingeing food because an entire package (four ½-cup servings) contains only 40 calories and 0 grams of carbohydrate. In contrast, *one* ½-cup serving of the sugary variety contains 80 calories and 19 grams of carbohydrate. The whole bowl (ouch!): 320 calories and 76 grams of carbohydrate.

Back to the sugar-free, jazz it up by combining two flavors: lemon and lime, raspberry and strawberry, cherry and cranberry. Substitute plain or flavored seltzer for the cold water. Or add small pieces of fresh or sugar-free frozen fruit or berries. For a patriotic, colorful dessert, prepare one of the red flavors and refrigerate about 1½ hours, or until thickened. Stir in fresh blueberries and refrigerate 4 hours, or until firm.

75 **HAVE A GUILTLESS BLT** ■ Pan-broil 3 strips of turkey bacon. Layer with a sliced tomato on a leaf of romaine. Wrap and eat. Approximately 90 calories, 6 grams carbohydrate, 9 grams protein, only 1.5 grams fat.

76 **CHOCOLATE FIX I: CHOCOLATE MILK** ■ Making your own chocolate syrup is a calorie and carbohydrate bargain. One brand's (2 tablespoon) serving of chocolate syrup has 100 calories, 25 grams of carbohydrate, 20 of them sugar. Another brand has 120 calories, 29 grams of carbohydrate, 23 of them sugar. Even a "lite" version has 50 calories, 12 grams of carbohydrate, 10 of them sugar.

My own chocolate syrup has 40 calories per 2-tablespoon serving, but only 6 grams of carbohydrate—no sugar. It also packs 2 grams of fiber into each serving. Put 2 tablespoons of plain (baking) cocoa into a large glass. Add 3 envelopes of Equal or a similar sweetener and 2–3 tablespoons of hot water. Stir well to make a syrup, add low-fat or skim milk, and stir again. Drink up guiltlessly!

You can also rev up this syrup with almond, rum, or cognac flavoring. Try it in your coffee for a very-low-calorie treat.

77 **CHECK FOOD LABELS BEFORE YOU BUY** ■ Little differences in calorie, carbohydrate, and fat between brands add up. One brand of garlic and herb pasta sauce has 110 calories per ½-cup serving, with 17 grams of carbohydrate, including 11 grams of sugar, 4 grams of fat, and 2 grams each of fiber and protein.

A "healthier" competitor has only 50 calories per ½-cup serving, with 11 grams of carbohydrate, including 8 grams of sugar, 0 grams of fat, and 3 grams each of fiber and protein: less than half the calories, two-thirds of the carbohydrates, and more fiber and protein.

78

CHOCOLATE FIX II: RUM OR COGNAC TRUFFLES ■ I created this recipe for my chocoholic diabetic and nondiabetic friends. The truffles' flavor is so incredibly intense that just one or two are luxuriously satisfying. And each truffle has only 3 grams of carbohydrate.

1 7 oz. bar Hershey's Special Dark Chocolate
5 oz. unsweetened baking chocolate
7 tbsp. heavy cream
3 tbsp. dark rum or cognac
approximately ½ cup raw almonds, chopped fine

- Break the chocolate into small pieces and place in large heat-proof bowl.
- In heavy saucepan, bring cream to just boiling and pour over chocolate. Let sit for 5 minutes, then stir until smooth.
- Add rum or cognac and stir again.
- Cover bowl and refrigerate 3 hours to overnight.
- With melon bailer, scoop and shape truffles, then roll in chopped almonds.
- Keep in covered container. Serve at room temperature.

YIELD: approximately 50 truffles; 60 calories and 3 grams carbohydrate per truffle.
VARIATION: Substitute Grand Marnier or Sabra liqueur for the rum or cognac, and add grated orange zest to the chopped almonds in which to roll the truffles. Approximately 70 calories and 4 grams carbohydrate per truffle.

79

MAGIC IN MUSHROOMS ■ I can't think of many foods that are as delicious and as low-calorie, low-carbohydrate, and low-fat as mushrooms. Most varieties of mushrooms contain less than 30 calories, 2 grams of carbohydrate, and only a trace of fat in a ½-cup portion.

Some mushrooms possess valuable medicinal properties, too. The Chinese mushroom known as the black tree ear has been proved to be an anticoagulant, similar to aspirin. It may help prevent narrowed arteries—a cause of high blood pressure—and clots that are a special concern for us diabetics.

Shiitake mushrooms contain lentinan, a strong antiviral substance that kills many viruses, stimulates the immune system, and lowers cholesterol when it is eaten daily.

80 QUICK GAZPACHO ■ Mix ½ cup "healthy" garlic and herb pasta sauce with ½ cup water. Chill. Top with diced red, yellow, or green pepper and/or chives and parsley.

Approximately 50 calories, 11 grams carbohydrate, 3 grams protein, 0 grams fat.

81 THE BEST TIME TO CHEAT ■ If you *do* cheat on your diet just a little, do it right after you exercise. Your metabolism will still be revved up, so you'll burn those extra calories and carbohydrates more quickly.

82 BE WARY OF "DIABETIC" COOKBOOKS ■ A helpful friend recently gave me a cookbook that had "sugar free" right in its title. However, a careful reading of the cover "explained" that the recipes used only "all-natural sweeteners."

What does this mean? Honey, date sugar, apple-juice concentrate, dried figs, brown-rice syrup, raisins—often more than one in the same recipe.

The per-serving data make it clear that most diabetics and dieters would shun this book. Most of the recipes contain around 200 calories and 30 grams of carbohydrate per serving; one recipe for Apple Spice Cake contained 295 calories and 38 grams of carbohydrate per 1" x 8" slice. That's roughly 20 percent of my daily calories and 30 percent of my daily carbohydrates. Of the more than 100 recipes in this cookbook, I found only a scant handful that met my calorie and carbohydrate requirements, so I gave the cookbook to my local library.

83 **LET YOURSELF SPLURGE ONCE A WEEK** ■ One of the most successful dieters I know has kept his weight loss for over twenty years. His secret? He watches his calories, carbohydrates, and fats six days a week, but on Saturday *or* Sunday, he lets himself feast a little. The next day, he's back to watching his food intake.

84 **CUT THE FAT, CUT THE CALORIES I** ■ Trim all fat off meat before broiling, roasting, or stewing it.

85 **CUT THE FAT, CUT THE CALORIES II** ■ Broil or roast meat in a ridged aluminum-foil pan. The meat will sit and cook on the ridges while the fat drains below, away from the meat.

86 **CUT THE FAT, CUT THE CALORIES III** ■ Blot broiled or roasted meat with a paper towel or napkin before serving it. See how much fat is absorbed? This little trick also works beautifully on your monthly slice of pizza.

87 **CHOOSE CHOPSTICKS TO SLOW DOWN** ■ Use chopsticks for all kinds of food—not just Asian cuisine. You'll benefit greatly from using them at home. Chopsticks slow down your eating speed, so you'll feel full faster on less food. And slowing down will give you the opportunity to taste and enjoy your food more.

Chopsticks also let you exercise your fingers and hands without realizing it, which can reduce the risks of carpal tunnel syndrome and arthritis.

As an added bonus, learning to master chopsticks will make you smile at yourself and at the world.

88 **LEARN A NEW RECIPE EVERY WEEK** ■ Diet and nutrition are a full-time "job" for everyone concerned with optimum health. You'll get more joy out of that job by turning it into a pleasurable hobby.

Find and tweak unusual recipes for chicken, fish, dairy, grains, and fruits and vegetables. Will they taste better with more or different herbs or spices? Sure, you'll have some results that you wouldn't repeat, but so do professional chefs. At the end of a year, you should have at least twenty healthy new recipes to feast on.

89 **TURN AN APPETIZER INTO DINNER** ■ This trick works especially well in hot weather, when you don't want to cook.

Supersize a shrimp or crabmeat cocktail for your main course. Start with 6–8 ounces of chilled boiled shrimp or a can of crabmeat on a bed of lettuce or greens and top with 2 tablespoons of cocktail sauce (approximately 10 calories, 3 grams carbohydrate). Add a slice of whole-grain bread, if you like. Finish your feast with fresh fruit or berries.

A cheese plate with fruit and whole-grain crackers is another excellent choice.

90 **DOWNSIZE YOUR PLATE SIZE** ■ Because you "eat with your eyes," a portion of food looks bigger if it's put on a smaller plate. In addition, you can't put as much food on a smaller plate.

Take advantage of this strategy by substituting a luncheon plate for your dinner plate. The average luncheon plate is 60 percent the size of the average dinner plate—47 square inches vs. 79 square inches—so you'll cut back on your food intake without really being conscious that you're doing it.

And no going back for seconds, except for salads or green and yellow veggies.

91 **OPEN-FACE YOUR SANDWICHES** ■ When you make your sandwich with one slice of bread instead of two, you save approximately 80 calories and—even more important—16 grams of carbohydrate.

Unless you are brown-bagging your sandwich, it's better to make and eat an *open* sandwich because it has the same surface size as the usual two-slice variety. However, if you're packing your sandwich, cut the slice of bread in half, make a thick half-sandwich, and eat it slowly.

92 **MAKE CHOCOLATE PART OF YOUR MEAL PLAN** ■ Chocolate lovers, rejoice! If you can stop at one or two pieces of chocolate, this tip is for you.

You probably already know the medical benefits of chocolate. It contains theobromine, a proven antidepressant, and resveratrol, the phytochemical in red wine that has been linked to a reduced risk of coronary disease and cancer.

Chocolate and a glass of 1% milk can be a good occasional lunch. Three blocks of a 7- or 8-ounce Hershey Special Dark, milk chocolate, or milk chocolate with almonds bar weigh 37 grams and "cost" 200 calories for the first two flavors and 210 calories for the almond variety. Carbohydrate grams range from 19 to 22, fat grams from 12 to 13, and protein grams from 2 to 4. The milk adds 100 calories, 12 grams of carbohydrate, 8 grams of protein, and only 2.5 grams of fat. Your total will be only 300–310 calories, with 31–34 grams of carbohydrate, 10–12 grams of protein, and 14–15 grams of fat.

This is *not* the kind of quickie meal to eat every day, but it provides enough nutritional and medical benefits to allow indulging in once or twice a week without feeling guilty.

93 **KNOW THE DIFFERENCE BETWEEN HUNGER AND THIRST** ■ It sounds very simple, but in fact many people reach for food when they are really thirsty.

Check this for yourself by drinking a glass of ice water when you think you are hungry. Wait five minutes. Do you feel less hungry now? If not, have a little snack.

94 **BEING A GOURMET WON'T WRECK YOUR BUDGET** ■ You can feast on very little money. Take the time to shop for the freshest food; it may mean going to three or four stores instead of one megasupermarket.

Pass up junk food, fast food, and prepared food. They are usually too high in calories, fat, carbohydrates, and sodium. They cost more than they are worth.

Instead, do your food shopping European-style. Spend time choosing perfect meat, fish, and produce. They will be fresher than at the supermarkets, which use regional distribution. Take advantage of seasonal bargains. Once in a while, splurge on the exotic, like raspberries in the winter or doughnut peaches. Turn your butcher and greengrocer into friends by asking their advice. Buy your whole-grain bread at the bakery on the morning they make it. Buy your rolls one at a time.

Aren't you worth all this extra work?

95 **PLAN MEALS IN ADVANCE . . .** ■ It's easier to eat right if you plan your meals in advance. Read store flyers to learn about weekly specials, make shopping lists, and try to shop only once or twice a week. It's much smarter to buy "family packs" of meat at bargain prices, and then wrap and freeze single portions.

Many busy people cook in batches on weekends and freeze individual-size portions, then just reheat and add a different salad or vegetable and dessert every night.

96 **BUT GIVE YOURSELF SOME LEEWAY** ■ Give yourself permission to be spontaneous, too. You may see some interesting food on display, or taste it in an in-store promotion, or even see it in another customer's grocery cart. Be flexible: If it intrigues you, buy it.

97 **JAZZ UP YOUR WATER WHEN IT GETS BORING** ■ Drinking those eight glasses of water day after day can become boring.

Change the taste by adding these flavorings:

- ◗ spearmint or peppermint extract.
- ◗ 1–2 tablespoons of orange, apple, or pineapple juice.
- ◗ almond extract. You can make a zero-calorie orzata (Italian almond syrup) with almond extract and aspartame.

Let these suggestions inspire you to experiment further!

98 **BRUSH YOUR TEETH AFTER EVERY MEAL** ■ If you brush or use a mouthwash, you'll be less inclined to eat again afterward.

99 **EXPERIMENT WITH HERBS AND SPICES** ■ Herbs and spices can completely change the taste of bland foods and enhance the flavor of others.

You are familiar with black and red pepper, but there are dozens of varieties. There are even subtle differences among different types of sea salt.

Experiment with the more unusual herbs, both fresh and dried. You may use six or eight frequently, but there are at least two or three dozen in many supermarkets. You'll get maximum flavor from buying whole spices like mustard, allspice, cloves, nutmeg, and pepper, and grinding them yourself as you need them. (Doing this will also perfume your home.)

Although you should avoid prepared herbs containing salt (buy minced or powdered onion or garlic instead of onion or garlic salt), there are many other interesting combinations. Mrs. Dash makes twelve different varieties—all salt-free.

100 **DITCH THE "I WAS GOOD/I WAS BAD" MIND-SET** ■ When you say to yourself or tell your friends, "I was good; I had fish and a salad for dinner yesterday." Or "I was bad; I had doughnuts for breakfast this morning," you are reverting to an emotional childhood, in which you are a good or bad kid out to either please or disobey Mommy or the latest authority figure: doctor, nutritionist, diabetes educator.

You have the power—not the authority figures, and certainly not the food. Instead of "good" or "bad," take the approach that if you over-ate at your last meal, you can eat less at the next one, and it will balance by the end of the day or the week. Every meal gives you a new opportunity to eat sensibly and healthfully.

101

CANCEL YOUR MEMBERSHIP IN THE CLEAN-PLATE CLUB ■ Our mothers may have taught us too well. They forced us to join the Clean Plate Club because children were starving in Europe or Asia or Africa, so we shouldn't waste our food. That was a sin, and they made us feel horribly guilty if we didn't eat every morsel.

Rise above that ancient guilt trip. You're an intelligent, independent adult now. It's better to waste money on food that you throw away than to spend it on doctors and drugs.

102

TAKE THE GLYCEMIC INDEX WITH A GRAIN OF SALT ■ The glycemic index is really an *average* obtained from the test results of many people. It is not a precise mathematical number.

"Average" means that some people with diabetes will react to a food with a high blood-glucose number, some with a low blood-glucose number, and most will fall somewhere in the middle. And many of those people will have significantly different blood-glucose numbers when they eat that food the next time, and the next.

Accordingly, many diabetics should pay more attention to the way individual high-carbohydrate foods affect *them,* as though they were having allergic reactions to those foods. For example, one of my insulin-dependent friends can eat a potato or one-half cup of rice, and his evening blood glucose will rise only 20–30 points, where another insulin-dependent friend's evening blood glucose will rise 70–80 points and will still be high the next morning.

103 BALANCE YOUR NUTRITION BY THE WEEK ■ You don't have to balance every single meal nutritionally. It may be more convenient to achieve balance over an entire week or longer. Especially if you live alone, you may find it easier to eat the same lunch or dinner two or three days in a row. When shrimp is on sale, you may enjoy eating shrimp marinara several days in a row, followed by grilled shrimp brochettes, followed by shrimp stir-fry or shrimp salad.

Next week, chicken, beef, or dairy may be on sale, and they will offer a basket of other nutritional benefits. Over a month, it all adds up and balances out.

104 LET YOUR BLOOD GLUCOSE READING DECIDE WHAT AND HOW MUCH YOU WILL EAT ■ Many successful diabetics base their meal plans on their blood-glucose readings. For example, if their reading is 70–100, they may have a larger portion of carbohydrates, if it is 120–140, they may have an average portion, and if it is over 250, they may have a smaller portion.

105 ENJOY FESTIVAL FOODS—BUT IN SMALL PORTIONS ■ Our lives would be very dreary without the foods we eat at celebrations: birthdays, weddings, sweet sixteens, bar and bas mitzvahs, confirmations, graduations, Thanksgivings, religious holidays.

It's OK to eat—and enjoy—a small piece of cake with friends and family—especially if you scrape off most of the frosting.

106 RESTAURANT SAVVY I: BECOME A "REGULAR" ■ Find a local restaurant you like and patronize it often. You'll get better, faster service—a blessing when your blood glucose is dropping. Having a regular waiter or waitress also guarantees solicitous treatment: "This is fresh," or "This isn't as good today."

107

RESTAURANT SAVVY II: ALWAYS ASK HOW A DISH IS MADE ■ Then ask questions like:

"Can you serve it with the sauce on the side?"

"Can it be sautéed or stir-fried instead of fried?"

"Can the chef make it without flour or cornstarch? Without the starchy vegetables? With more mushrooms and peppers?"

108

RESTAURANT SAVVY III: DOGGIE-BAG STRATEGY ■ Of course, given the generous restaurant servings, you'll try to eat only half, and have the rest packed up for you in a doggie bag.

Realistically, though, many of us still get seduced into cleaning our plates. To avoid overeating, bring your own little covered plastic bowl and put half your entree into the bowl immediately. Then you can eat the rest and scrape your plate clean with a clear conscience.

109

RESTAURANT SAVVY IV: ORDER OFF THE MENU ■ You can do this most easily if you're a regular at that restaurant.

At your local Chinese restaurant, for example, you can create your own dish:

"Can your chef mix breast of chicken with shrimp? In a brown sauce without flour or cornstarch? How about with shredded ginger? Tree ears? Black mushrooms? Sweet red and yellow peppers?"

Be a Cantonese Escoffier! The sky's the limit, and your new creation will be loaded with vitamins and minerals.

110

RESTAURANT SAVVY V: BRING RESTAURANT IDEAS HOME ■ Just as you bring your ideas to a favorite restaurant for execution, adapt a restaurant's dishes and presentations for home use.

It can be as simple as a garnish, or which fresh or dried herbs are used to embellish a dish. The unusual ingredients of a fresh fruit salad.

Seasonings. (Many years later, I still remember the marvelous broiled grapefruit at the Chalet Suzanne in Lake Wales, Florida.)

Professional chefs have created these unusual dishes and presentations. Copying them can bring you kudos at home.

111 GOT THE MUNCHIES? GO FOR "FIDDLE" FOOD ■

"Fiddle" food is food that you have to fiddle with before you can eat it. You have to take it out of its shell, cut it up, unwrap it. That's going to slow down how much you eat. The best examples are nuts—especially almonds, walnuts, and Brazil nuts, which really take some work. Bonus: Unshelled nuts are also fresher and more nutritious.

Or try cutting up a whole fresh pineapple and nibbling on it instead of buying it already cut up.

112 NAVIGATE THE CARBOHYDRATE CONTROVERSY ■

The American Diabetes Association's diet emphasizes carbohydrates. It urges us to get 50 to 60 percent of our calories from carbohydrates, which break down into sugars. The ADA Web site tells us to make starches "the centerpiece of the meal."

The ADA is not alone in its advice. Boston's prestigious Joslin Diabetes Center recommends that 45 to 60 percent of our calories come from carbohydrates. Here's the breakdown, using the ADA's 55 percent yardstick:

DAILY

CALORIES	CHO	BREAKFAST	LUNCH	DINNER	SNACK
			GRAMS		
1,200	165	33	58	58	17
1,500	206	41	72	72	21
1,800	248	50	87	87	25
2,100	289	58	101	101	29

Critics of these recommended high-carbohydrate diets are vocal. Among them are physicians who have diabetes. According to Dr. Richard Bernstein, a Type 1 diabetic for nearly sixty years, people whose bodies can't process carbohydrates should not be told by the diabetic establishment to eat a diet that is mostly sugar.

Admittedly, Bernstein's regimen is tough for many of us to follow. It limits carbohydrates to 6 grams for breakfast and 12 grams each for lunch and for dinner. Nonetheless, many people have had amazing success with it and have had normal test results for years.

Bernstein is not alone in his criticism. Diabetes specialist Lois Jovanovic calls the ADA high-carbohydrate diet "malpractice," because "diabetes is a disease of carbohydrate intolerance."

A Harvard Medical School study found that the current food pyramid—"fats bad, carbohydrates good"—is backward and can actually increase the risk of heart attack, obesity, and stroke.

How do *you* sort out the controversy? Logic seems to be on the side of Drs. Bernstein and Jovanovic and the Harvard Medical School. If you have gyrating blood-sugar readings and unacceptable lab results, consider trying to restrict your daily carbohydrates to 30 grams or, if that's too difficult, to 60 grams, for one month. *If* you and your doctor are happy with the results, stay with your new low-carbohydrate eating plan.

113 **FOR PIZZA LOVERS** ■ Don't give up your favorite pizza, just ditch the dough. Even thin-crust pizzas can contain 10–15 grams of carbohydrate in the crust per slice.

Pick up your fork and enjoy the pizza topping, which has much more flavor. You can probably have two slices' worth if you skip the crust.

114 **ENJOY THE CRUNCH OF RAW FOOD** ■ There's a serious kick in foods with texture. In addition to carrot and celery sticks, try strips of sweet peppers, green beans, and even asparagus stalks.

Explore the dozens of varieties of apples and pears developed specifically for eating (rather than cooking). A piece of fruit and a wedge or two of cheese can make an easy, nutritious meal.

115 BURN CALORIES WITH ICE WATER ■ Drinking ice water has a benefit beyond hydrating you and cooling you off. Your body must burn calories to bring the ice water up to your body temperature—as much as 200 calories a day.

116 BUY AT FARM STANDS AND FARMERS' MARKETS ■ For freshness and variety, farm stands and farmers' markets are your best bets. Most large cities now offer farmers' markets at least once a week.

Farms and orchards where you can pick your own berries and fruits are another great choice. The bending and stretching will also exercise you, and picking berries and fruit is a wonderful education for your kids.

117 GROW YOUR OWN ■ Better yet, grow your own! Even if all you have is a kitchen window, you can grow your own herbs. Rosemary, basil, and tarragon are good choices.

More room? A planter on a terrace, a backyard patch, or a little piece of a community garden will give you enough room for at least one or two raspberry bushes, encircled by strawberry plants. (Gardeners call this doubling-up tactic "underplanting." It lets you utilize every square inch of room.) Tomatoes need lots of space, but you can usually grow patio tomatoes in a planter.

More space in warmer climates will let you grow vegetables and fruit trees.

Nothing is more fun than picking your own food and eating it right away!

118 GO GARLIC! ■ Many of us feel that garlic should be elevated to its own food group. Besides tasting marvelous and being the soul food of many ethnic groups, garlic has many medical benefits. It lowers blood pressure and is an anticoagulant and a powerful antibiotic. It also boosts the immune system.

119

"SUGAR-FREE" IS NOT CARBOHYDRATE-FREE ■ You probably already know that high-fructose corn syrup and glucose—two common ingredients in processed foods—are not considered "sugar" for the purposes of food labeling, but can drive your blood glucose into the stratosphere. Honey isn't as common an ingredient because it's much more expensive.

Sugar alcohols are an ingredient that many people with diabetes are not as familiar with. Most of them discover that sugar alcohol makes their blood-glucose levels zoom, so they read food labels carefully and avoid foods made with it.

120

THE BENEFITS OF BREAKFAST ■ Your mother was right. Breakfast is the most important meal of the day. Your body has been without food for approximately 12 hours, which means that your rate of burning calories has slowed down. If you make lunch your first meal, then your metabolic rate has dropped for 18 hours. Harvard Medical School researchers found that breakfast eaters have one-half the risk of developing obesity and insulin resistance, which is a major risk factor for diabetes and heart disease, compared with people who skip breakfast.

Other studies show that people who eat breakfast eat less fat and fewer high-calorie foods all day. They are also less likely to overeat at night.

121

BREAKFAST ON THE GO ■ You can make yourself a grab-and-go breakfast in less than five minutes.

Put 1 cup of plain lowfat yogurt in a small container. If desired, mix in 1–2 teaspoons of fruit spread.

Or take a small wedge of your favorite cheese or ½ cup of lowfat cottage cheese.

Add an apple or an orange and a travel mug of coffee or tea. Now you can breakfast at your desk.

122 **SALAD DRESSING SMARTS I: THE SMALL-PORTION SOLUTION** ■ According to the labels on the bottles, 2 tablespoons constitutes a portion. That means horrendously high calorie, carbohydrate, and fat counts—often 160–170 calories per portion, which equals 10 percent of many diabetics' daily allowance.

However, you can cut back on that 2-tablespoon portion easily. If you limit yourself to 1 or 2 *teaspoons* of your favorite salad dressing, you'll be consuming only 17 to 33 percent of those calories, carbohydrates, and fats.

123 **SALAD DRESSING SMARTS II: POUR OFF THE OIL** ■ Many bottled salad dressings are made with oil that rises to the top. Cut the calories and fat and intensify the flavor by pouring off at least half the oil as soon as you open the bottle. (Then refrigerate immediately after use, of course.)

124 **SALAD DRESSING SMARTS III: DILUTE THE FAT AND CALORIES** ■ If your favorite salad dressing is a ranch or creamy type, dilute it with an equal quantity of lowfat buttermilk. You'll still have the zesty flavor, but you'll cut the calories and fat.

125 **SALAD DRESSING SMARTS IV: SKINNY-DIP!** ■ What's a salad without dressing? Cow food, boring and maybe even tasteless. To solve this problem, when you get your low-calorie, low-fat salad dressing on the side, dip your fork into the dressing *before* spearing the greens. You'll use a lot less dressing this way, so you'll get almost all the taste, but avoid almost all the calories and fat.

126 **BEEFY BONUS** ■ You can feel good about eating beef. Lean beef packs a powerful nutritional punch. It delivers three times more iron, six times more zinc, and eight times more vitamin B_{12} than a skinless chicken breast.

127 **FEAST ON HOMEMADE NUT BUTTERS** ■ Do you love peanut butter but want to avoid those nasty hydrogenated oils and trans fats? Make your own!

All you need is a blender or food processor, dry-roasted unsalted peanuts, and about five minutes.

You can also make almond or cashew butter with raw nuts, or toast them first in the oven.

Once you make nut butters at home, you'll never want store-bought again.

128 **MAKE YOUR OWN NO-CARBOHYDRATE MAPLE SYRUP** ■ Many of us miss having maple syrup on their weekend low-carbohydrate French toast or pancakes. The real thing is too high in carbohydrates and calories and can wreck your blood-glucose numbers.

Try this instead. Use maple extract straight from the bottle or dilute it with water. Add aspartame if it's not sweet enough. Pour and enjoy!

129 **KEEP FAT IN YOUR DIET** ■ There are many good reasons to keep some fat in your diet.

Fat causes your body to produce the smallest amount of insulin. Replacing dietary fat with carbohydrates actually causes higher insulin levels, and that will increase your body fat and can lead to obesity.

Fat also stops carbohydrate cravings. It satisfies our hunger longer, so we are less tempted to eat. A few grams of fat per day can wind up saving hundreds of calories a day in food intake.

130 **START YOUR DIET ON SATURDAY** ■ We're all familiar with the "I'll start my diet on Monday" syndrome. The problem is that we then act like condemned criminals facing their last meals and pig out. After all, we'll start a rigorous diet tomorrow.

The result is that we lose two days and usually put on five pounds. And we start the week beating up on ourselves.

Saturday can be an easier day to start your diet. You are usually not as rushed and can linger over a well-planned breakfast, lunch, and dinner. You can even do some gourmet cooking for the rest of the week.

By Monday, you will have gotten a head start on your diet. And you'll probably weigh less, too.

131 ICE-CREAM CALORIES AND CARBOHYDRATES VARY GREATLY ■ Ice-cream calories and carbohydrates can vary by over 100 percent per portion. For example, a ½-cup portion of Breyer's coffee ice cream has 140 calories and 14 grams of carbohydrate, easy for diabetics and dieters alike to fit into their meal plans. But the same size portion of superpremium Godiva Chocolate Raspberry Truffle ice cream contains 290 calories and 32 grams of carbohydrate, which can really capsize your diet.

132 UNDERSTAND YOUR EMOTIONAL EATING ■ Many people eat for reasons that have nothing to do with physical hunger. They may be angry, anxious, bored, lonely, or sad.

It's not easy, and it can be painful, but try to find the reason you are eating (usually, overeating) and deal with it. Confide your feelings to a journal, then call a friend or go for a walk, rent a movie, or tune in to the Cartoon Network or Comedy Central.

133 DIETING? ATKINS MAY WORK BETTER THAN OTHER PLANS ■ A recent Harvard research study found that people on low-carbohydrate diets, like the Atkins plan, ate more than those on an American Heart Association low-fat diet—and still lost weight.

This news comes as no surprise to many of us diabetics who thrive on limiting our carbohydrates, rather than counting every calorie.

134 CUSTOMIZE YOUR WEIGHT-LOSS PLAN ■ In dieting, one size does *not* fit all. We all have our favorite foods

and hated foods, carbohydrate foods that raise our blood-glucose readings horrendously and those that don't. Some of us fare better on three meals a day, and some with four or five smaller meals.

Find a plan that works for *you*. It may take weeks of trial and error, but what counts is your long-term success in losing weight and keeping it off.

135
WORK YOUR FAVORITE FOODS INTO YOUR WEIGHT-LOSS PLAN ■ You can prevent binge eating by including your favorite foods in your weight-loss or eating plan.

One of my diabetic friends, who is a diabetes educator, says, "I'll work out at the gym in order to have ice cream." Most of us would agree.

Even without the workout, you can plan for a small dish of ice cream or two small bonbons or a piece of fruit for dessert every night without exceeding your carbohydrate quota. And that little treat can satisfy you enough to keep you on your diet the rest of the time.

136
SUBSTITUTE SPRAY FOR SHORTENING ■ Do the math, and you'll become a convert.

One tablespoon of oil contains 122 calories, one tablespoon of butter or margarine, 104 calories. But a one-second spritz of cooking spray—enough to coat an omelet pan or skillet—contains only 7 calories.

Cooking sprays come in several flavors, like butter, olive oil, lemon, and garlic.

137
UNDERSTAND THE BMI ■ The Body Mass Index (BMI) is a convenient number that expresses the ratio of your weight to your height as a single number.

To calculate it, multiply your weight in pounds by 703. Divide this number by your height in inches, and then divide it again by your height in inches.

Thus, someone who is 5' 5" tall and weighs 160 pounds has a BMI of 26.6. A BMI under 18.5 is considered underweight, 18.5–24.9 is considered normal, 25.0–29.9 is considered overweight, and over 30.0 is considered obese.

However, there are limitations to this easy-to-understand number. The most common is that serious bodybuilders may have BMIs between 25 and 30, but not be overweight because muscle tissue weighs more than fat.

138 **ENJOY YOUR WINE!** ■ You may have heard of "the French paradox," which suggests that the French consumption of wine offsets the fat in their diet and helps prevent coronary disease and cancer.

Here's the science behind it: Wine—especially red wine—contains large quantities of resveratrol, a phytochemical that has been linked to a reduced risk or coronary disease and cancer. Some plants, fruits, seeds, and other grape products contain resveratrol, too, but not as high a concentration, and many of them are high in carbohydrates.

A glass of dry red wine at dinner offers other benefits, too. It aids digestion and slows down your eating. You may actually eat less and enjoy it more! And dry red wine also increases HDL (good) cholesterol in some people.

139 **COOK WITH IT, TOO** ■ Cooking with wine adds flavor, but not calories. That's because heat evaporates the alcohol, so all you are left with is the taste.

The increased flavor also lets you reduce less beneficial ingredients, like fat or oil and salt.

Cooking with liquors like cognac, rum, and bourbon, doesn't add calories, either, but sweet liqueurs like amaretto and Grand Marnier should be used sparingly because of their high caloric and carbohydrate content.

140 **JUMP-START YOUR DIET WITH A FAST** ■ Admittedly, this strategy isn't for everyone; but a one- or two-day fast won't hurt most adults, and should pay off in a weight loss of approximately five pounds.

Please check first with your doctor.

You must also:

Drink at least six 8-ounce glasses of water per day.

Adjust your insulin so that you are taking only your basal dosage, not the dose or type of insulin that you need for meal coverage.

141

MAKE COTTAGE CHEESE MORE EXCITING ■ Lovely, bland cottage cheese is a dieter's friend. (But it's not always a diabetic's friend. Dr. Bernstein says it increases blood glucose a lot in some of his patients. One trick to reduce the lactose content is to wash it before you use it.) The 2 percent fat variety contains 90 calories, 6 grams of carbohydrate, 2.5 grams of fat, and 12 grams of protein per ½-cup serving, and the 1 percent variety contains only 80 calories, 4 grams of carbohydrate, 1 gram of fat, and 14 grams of protein.

But this diet buddy can get a little boring after a while.

Go spicy or sweet to perk up your interest without boosting your calorie or carbohydrate intake.

Spicy: Add freeze-dried chives or onions (nice and crunchy!), garlic powder, chopped hot or sweet peppers, a teaspoon of salad dressing, salsa, or mustard.

Sweet: Add vanilla, almond, orange, lemon, or peppermint extracts, with or without sugar substitute.

142

EAT SPINACH AT LEAST THREE TIMES A WEEK ■ Spinach can help prevent two eye diseases that diabetics are especially susceptible to: cataracts and age-related macular degeneration.

Spinach is loaded with folate and the phytochemicals lutein and zeaxanthin, both of which are found in the macula (central portion) of the retina. Zeaxanthin has been linked to a lower risk of age-related macular degeneration, the leading cause of blindness in people over the age of fifty-five. Zeaxanthin is also believed to protect against the development of cataracts.

Maybe Popeye was right!

Note: Orange peppers also have a high zeaxanthin and lutein content, but they are seasonal and often expensive.

143 **WEIGHT-Y MATTERS** ■ It makes more sense to weigh yourself once a week than every single day.

Even if you weigh yourself at the same time every morning (after the bathroom and before breakfast), your weight can still fluctuate by 2–3 pounds from day to day.

If you weigh yourself only once a week, these little increases and decreases smooth out, and you get a more accurate reading.

However, if you are obsessive and *must* weigh yourself every morning, keep track of your daily numbers in a notebook and divide by 7 once a week to calculate your average weight.

144 **SUBSTITUTE SPAGHETTI SQUASH FOR PASTA** ■ Plain pasta is high in carbohydrates, the bane of many people with diabetes. One cup of cooked regular or whole-wheat spaghetti, for example, contains approximately 198 calories and 41 grams of carbohydrate. But one cup of spaghetti squash contains only 46 calories and 10 grams of carbohydrate. Spaghetti squash is also an excellent source of folic acid and fiber and ecintributes some potassium and a small amount of vitamin A.

Mangia!

145 **WHEN YOU *MUST* BAKE** ■ Sometimes we all get the urge to bake. It's OK to give in to that warm, nurturing desire if you plan ahead to prevent potential binge eating. Here's what you can do:

Invite one or more friends for coffee and that fresh-baked goodie. Give them any leftovers to take home.

Eat one and freeze the rest.

Or eat one and bring the rest to an older neighbor or to a nursing home.

146 **CINNAMON BUN SUBSTITUTE** ■ Breakfast pastries have been supersized to mammoth proportions. A

Cinnabon weighs 7.5 ounces and contains 670 calories—nearly half the daily allowance for most of us—and 12 teaspoons of sugar and 34 grams of fat. The Pecanbon is even worse: 1,100 calories and 56 grams of fat.

But you can get a cinnamon-bun taste without all the calories, carbohydrates, and fat.

Take a slice of whole-wheat bread, spread with a thin layer of butter or margarine, sprinkle with cinnamon and a sugar substitute like Equal or Splenda. Warm in the microwave and eat. Total calories approximately 100, with 13 grams of carbohydrate and less than 3 grams of fat.

147 **CINNAMON BOOSTS THE EFFECT OF INSULIN ▪** Just ¼ teaspoon of cinnamon a day increases the effect of the insulin that your body produces or that you inject. Scientists at the USDA Human Nutrition Research Center discovered that methylhydroxy chalcone polymer (MHCP)—the active chemical in cinnamon—makes insulin twenty times more active.

148 **OTHER HERBS AND SPICES WORK, TOO ▪** Allspice, nutmeg, and oregano also make insulin more active. They increase the effect of insulin more than eight times.

Of these, oregano is the least expensive and the easiest to add to your daily menu. It goes well with fresh tomatoes and tomato sauces, and you can even grow it on your windowsill.

149 **YO-YO DIETING IS HARMFUL ▪** You lose weight. You gain it back. You lose weight. You gain it back. Each time it's harder to lose the weight, and you may gain back even more, and more quickly.

This repeated pattern, called "yo-yo dieting," is dangerous. In its infinite wisdom, your body senses each successive diet as an attempt to starve it. Your body defends itself by slowing down your metabolism. Your body will actually try to increase its fat deposits to protect itself, and this can lead to cardiovascular disease and stroke.

150

HOW TO TREAT YOUR "THRIFTY GENE" ■ The "thrifty gene" theory explains our species' survival in the face of millennia of famine and disease. Historically, many population groups have survived times when food was scarce and uncertain because some of them were able to slow their metabolism and live on very few calories. Those people lived to pass on their "thrifty gene" to successive generations. It is Darwin's "survival of the fittest" in action.

Fast-forward to the present. Rather than hunting and gathering or growing our food and fearing famine, most of our hunting is for the nearest parking space in the supermarket lot. Now food is readily available, but our genes haven't learned that.

By adolescence or young adulthood, most of us know whether we possess the thrifty gene. We have learned through bitter experience how difficult it is for us to lose even five or ten pounds while our friends brag about how much they can eat without gaining weight.

How do you deal with your thrifty gene? Try these three strategies:

First, bring balance and sanity into your life by recognizing that you have a thrifty gene. You may never become an athlete or wear a size 6, but you should survive the next famine or Ice Age.

Second, avoid gaining any more weight. Lose weight slowly—over years, not weeks. Crash dieting will only make your thrifty gene more thrifty.

Third, increase your activity level. Try the tips in Chapter 5, "Exercise."

151

SNACKS CAN HELP YOU LOSE WEIGHT ■ You may be more successful with an eating plan that offers a mid-morning and a midafternoon snack. The logic is that you will not overeat at meals and so will actually eat less overall.

Typical "good" snacks are skinless turkey or chicken, low-fat cheese, hard-boiled eggs, vegetables, and small quantities of raw fruit.

152

AND SO CAN OATMEAL—MAYBE ■ Eating oatmeal for breakfast can also curb hunger and speed weight loss—but I admit to having some questions about the enthusiastic findings of a recent study. When scientists compared people who ate 350 calories of dry cereal to those who ate 350 calories of oatmeal, they found that the oatmeal eaters ate 30 percent less for lunch and also felt less hungry during the day.

My issue is that the study apparently compared a breakfast of 3 cups of dry cereal to 3 cups of oatmeal, but most people eat only 1 cup. In addition, those 3 cups of oatmeal contain 81 grams of carbohydrate—far too high a load for most people with diabetes to consume in a single meal.

Will oatmeal curb *your* appetite and help you lose weight? It may be worth a try in a smaller portion—especially for its high fiber and protein content.

153 HOT STUFF ■ Your love of spicy food can help you lose weight. Researchers found that when people ate a red sauce made with capsaicin—the phytochemical that makes chili peppers hot—they ate 200 fewer calories over the next three hours than when the sauce did not contain capsaicin.

154 KNOW YOUR DIETING STYLE ■ Do you prefer to weigh or measure your food? To count calories or carbohydrates? To eat meals or to graze? The closer your dieting plan comes to matching your usual eating pattern, the more likely it is that you will stick to your diet and lose weight.

155 GIVE YOURSELF "WIGGLE ROOM" ■ Whether or not you are dieting, your weight fluctuates every day. A range of three to five pounds is quite normal.

Give yourself some leeway. Don't be concerned as long as your weight stays within that five-pound range. But if your weight rises *above* that limit, it's time to diet more seriously.

156 **BELTS BEAT SCALES** ■ Dieting? Is the needle on your scale stuck? Try on a belt. Sometimes it takes a week or two before your scale shows a weight loss. But during that time your waistline will start shrinking, and your belt will show you that it has.

Keep on using that belt to check your progress. Especially when your weight hits a plateau and you become depressed, having to cinch your belt tighter will show you that your diet is really working.

157 **KNIT OR CROCHET** ■ Why is this tip in this chapter? Because knitting and crocheting can help you lose weight. Not only do they keep your fingers busy and away from food, but the clicking of the knitting needles and the in-and-out movement of the crochet hook are repetitive actions that can soothe you and send you into another, relaxing "zone."

Football great Rosey Grier made it acceptable for men to do needlepoint, so why shouldn't they try knitting or crocheting? A scarf is a great beginner's project because it needs no shaping and its finished measurements can be off by several inches and it won't be obvious.

158 **SALAD-BAR PITFALLS** ■ Salad bars can be perilous. The greens are great, but portion control and avoiding all the add-ons can be a problem. Steer clear of bacon chips, croutons, the dressings, some of which are loaded with calories, and the crackers and bread that are often served with them.

If you like the convenience and variety that salad bars offer, load up on the greens and raw vegetables, and spoon out the dressing parsimoniously.

159 **BROWN-BAG YOUR LUNCH** ■ When you bring your lunch from home, you are lured less by the ubiquitous fast-food restaurants and takeouts, and by nearby candy and soda machines.

Go gourmet with your own mixture of low-fat plain yogurt and diced fresh fruit or berries. Make salmon, crabmeat, or shrimp salad the night before, or eat them unadorned, out of the can. Eat raw veggies as finger food, with or without a *teaspoon* of salad dressing. (You can be more lavish with mustard.)

160 BREAK YOUR BINGE ■ Even the most dedicated dieter is bound to binge once every few months. Here are some ways to deal with this problem:

If you really, truly binge only once in a very great while, give yourself permission to do so, and adjust your medication—if necessary—the next time you check your blood glucose. *But* be honest with yourself about how often this habit occurs. Set a kitchen timer for five or ten minutes and *stop eating when the bell rings.*

If you binge more frequently, be aware of what triggers this behavior. The simplest fix is removing yourself from the "scene of the crime." Get out of your house and go for a walk. Visit a friend.

A stronger strategy comes from practitioners of aversion therapy. Place a thick rubber band over your wrist. It should fit snugly, like a bracelet. When you find yourself bingeing, snap the rubber band on the underside of your wrist—it should hurt—and say "Stop!" to yourself. Repeat if necessary.

161 UNDERDRESSING BURNS MORE CALORIES ■ Dress in lighter clothes than you need—you should feel a little cold, but not uncomfortably so—and your body thermostat has to work harder to maintain your temperature. That means burning more calories—about 5 percent more. You may also move more briskly to keep warm, and that will burn even more calories.

162 APPLE PIE SUBSTITUTE I ■ Sautéed apples can satisfy your taste for apple pie. But where a slice of apple pie contains 405 calories, 60 grams of carbohydrate, and 18 grams of fat, and a 3-ounce "snack pie" contains 266 calories, 33 grams of carbohydrate, and 14 grams of fat, this recipe contains only between 80 and 100 calories (depending on the size of the apple), 21 grams of carbohydrate, and less than 2 grams of fat—scarcely more than in a raw apple.

For each serving, peel and core one apple and cut it into 8–10 pieces. Spray a large skillet heavily with butter-flavored cooking spray and, if desired, 1 teaspoon butter. Add apple, stir, turn heat down, cover, and cook for 10 minutes. Sprinkle with 1 tablespoon Equal or Splenda and 1 teaspoon cinnamon. Raise heat to medium. Cook, stirring frequently, until apples are glazed—approximately 10 minutes. Serve hot or warm.

163

APPLE PIE SUBSTITUTE II ■ Baked apples are another tasty treat. This recipe, too, contains only about 20 calories more than a raw apple.

Preheat oven to 350 degrees. For each serving, take a large apple and core and peel the top half, leaving the bottom end intact. Dip the peeled portion in a mixture of 1 tablespoon lemon juice and 10 table-spoons water to prevent browning.

Place the apple in a baking dish with approximately ½" of water. Dilute ½ teaspoon no-sugar-added raspberry or apricot fruit spread with ½ teaspoon of water and spread on top of apple. Bake approximately 40 minutes.

Then fill the cavity of the apple with 1 teaspoon of the fruit spread and bake an additional 10 minutes. Serve hot or warm.

164

LIGHTEN YOUR BEER ■ The new "lite" and "ultralite" beers are a godsend to diabetics who love their brew. New brewing technologies have kept the flavor, but cut the calories and carbohydrates by one-third to one-half. Brewers will certainly keep on making their beers and ales more attractive to dieters, so keep on checking labels and Web sites for the latest new liquids.

165

USE YOGURT CHEESE INSTEAD OF CREAM CHEESE ■ You'll need a little advance planning (like the night before), a funnel, and a coffee filter. Your reward is a freshly made cheese that can be used like cream cheese or Neufchatel, with only a fraction of the calories and fat.

Preparation takes less than three minutes. Place the coffee filter in the funnel and suspend it in a glass or small bowl. Then fill the filter with plain low-fat yogurt, cover with plastic wrap, and refrigerate overnight. Discard the whey (liquid). Use the resulting cheese au naturel, blend fresh or dried herbs and garlic into it, or add vanilla or other flavoring extracts. Or you can substitute it for cream cheese in recipes.

Here's the caloric breakdown: One ounce of regular or whipped cream cheese contains 100 calories, 1 gram of carbohydrate, 10 grams of fat, and 2 grams of protein. Calculating the calories, carbohydrates, and fat content of yogurt cheese is a little less precise because of the speed at which the whey drains out of the yogurt and because there are no calculations for the whey itself.

However, ¼ cup of plain low-fat yogurt contains only 35 calories, 4 grams of fat, and 2.7 grams of protein. Furthermore, the whey, which is discarded, is a rich source of lactose (milk sugar), so the yogurt cheese you make probably contains less than 1 gram of carbohydrate.

166 BE HONEST WITH YOURSELF ■ Recently I ran into an acquaintance and was shocked to see that he had gained thirty pounds (about 20 percent of his body weight) in less than a year. When I asked him what had happened, he told me that he was now driving a cab twelve hours a day and living on fast food, like buying and devouring three hamburgers one after the other, or a box of doughnuts or a pizza.

"Why don't you buy five or six burgers and eat the meat and toss the buns?" I asked him.

"Well, I can't," he said evasively.

"Why don't you bring cheese slices, a couple of apples from home? You can eat lots of good food with one hand."

He didn't have a good answer for this, either.

He wasn't being honest with me, and I doubt that he is honest with himself. That will be his first step in planning to lose weight.

167 **FAST-FOOD RESTAURANTS MAY BE WORTH A SECOND LOOK** ■ After too many years, fast-food restaurants are finally offering low-carbohydrate, low-fat dishes that we can eat. Chains like Applebee's, Burger King, McDonald's, Ruby Tuesday, and Wendy's have all added grilled chicken, main-course salads, steamed vegetables, and other nutritious entrees to boost their business among health-conscious consumers. These good-for-you choices are usually highlighted or starred, which makes the menus easier to navigate.

168 **CHOOSE YOUR BREAD WISELY** ■ Most varieties of bread contain approximately the same number of calories and grams of carbohydrate per slice. But their glycemic index can differ greatly, which means that some varieties will not make your blood glucose zoom as much as others will.

The fineness or coarseness of the flour and the bread make a big difference in how rapidly your body breaks down the bread into glucose. The best breads for us diabetics are made of oats (kernels or bran) or rye. Rye, which includes pumpernickel, is especially nutritious, as it contains more protein, phosphorus, iron, potassium, and B vitamins and 3.5 times as much soluble fiber as wheat bread. Sourdough rye bread has one of the lowest glycemic-index and glycemic-load values of all breads.

169 **ADDING ACID CAN LOWER YOUR BLOOD GLUCOSE** ■ Researchers have found that a small amount of lemon juice or vinegar as an ingredient in salad dressing lowered blood glucose significantly. As little as 4 teaspoons of vinaigrette (4 teaspoons vinegar, 2 teaspoons oil) eaten in a salad at lunch or dinner lowered blood glucose by as much as 30 percent.

Lemon juice was found to be just as effective, so consider a glass or two of homemade cold or hot lemonade. And, as other acids can also lower your blood glucose, you may want to try sourdough bread, which contains both lactic and propionic acids, and that has been shown to reduce blood-glucose levels by 22 percent compared to white bread.

170
GRISLY FANTASIES MAY MOTIVATE YOU TO LOSE WEIGHT ■ Some people are more motivated by rewards, some by the possibility of punishment. If you respond more to the latter, think of the terrible things that can happen to you if you do not lose your excess weight and control your blood glucose better.

The possibility of having toes, feet, or legs amputated, of going blind, of needing a kidney transplant or going on dialysis may be frightening enough to make you decide to take action to improve your health.

171
DIETER'S MANTRA ■ When you are considering eating something, ask yourself: Is this really worth all the calories, carbohydrates, and fat?" Reciting this mantra will give you perspective: "A minute on my lips, a year on my hips."

172
NO-CARBOHYDRATE LUNCHES BOOST AFTERNOON ALERTNESS ■ Eating a no-carbohydrate lunch of lean meat or fish and salad or green vegetables helps you avoid the common afternoon slump. Here's why it works: Cutting carbohydrates prevents the release of serotonin, a brain chemical that can relax you to the point of sleep. But protein raises your level of dopamine, a brain chemical that boosts your alertness and also produces feelings of intense well-being.

173
FIND A DIET BUDDY ■ A friendly sense of competition can help both you and a friend lose weight.

Choose the same morning of the week to strip down to your skivvies and weigh in. Keep track of your starting weights in a small notebook, and use the same scale every week, for consistency. Bet no more than $5 or $10 per week, and the winner is the one who has lost the greatest percentage of weight that week. Keep up this little game for at least ten weeks, and you'll both be winners!

174 **BELT UP BEFORE YOU PARTY** ■ Are you going to a party where there will be lots of food and drink? Make a belt part of your outfit and cinch it snugly, or wear it under your clothing. Your suddenly tight belt will tell you that you couldn't—or shouldn't—eat another bite.

175 **GET NUTTY I** ■ Unsalted nuts are good for you! They are rich in protein, minerals, fiber, vitamin E and B vitamins, including folic acid, and healthful monounsaturated fats. Walnuts are especially rich in these good oils, but almonds contain nearly three times as much fiber.

176 **A DAILY EGG CAN BE SAFE** ■ The bad news: One egg contains 215 milligrams of cholesterol, two-thirds of the daily maximum.

The good news: Saturated fat plays a larger role in raising our blood cholesterol, and eggs contain very little saturated fat. So if your cholesterol is low and you are not at risk for heart disease, you can probably enjoy a daily egg, low in calories and high in protein and iron.

177 **BUTTER? MARGARINE?** ■ Margarine that is made from hydrogenated oil contains trans fats, which are as bad for your heart as the saturated fat in butter. Some newer margarines do not contain trans fats, and some contain a cholesterol-lowering ingredient. If you eat small amounts of butter or margarine (less than 1 teaspoon per day) and are on a healthy, balanced diet, it really doesn't matter whether you choose margarine or butter. Go for the taste you prefer.

178

WHEN PROCESSED IS BETTER THAN FRESH ■ In most cases, fresh fruit and vegetables are better for you than processed. But there is one major exception. Cooked and processed tomatoes contain lycopene—a phytochemical like beta carotene—that is more readily utilized by the body. In fact, ounce for ounce, tomato sauce, paste, or juice contain two to ten times as much available lycopene as fresh tomatoes.

179

GO FOR THE *DARK* GREEN . . . AND RED ■ The darkest-colored fruits and vegetables have more vitamins and minerals than their lighter-colored cousins. Besides, the darker plant pigments themselves may protect against chronic disease because they contain high levels of antioxidants. Choose kale, spinach, or romaine over iceberg lettuce, yams over white potatoes, red grapes over green.

180

CHECK PACKAGE LABELS FOR REFORMULATION ■ You may have decided to buy a packaged food based on its attractive nutritional numbers in a magazine or newspaper article.

But don't stop there—do a little more research. Especially if you cut out that article a while back "for future reference," as many of us do, check the package label against the article. Ingredients may have been added or subtracted, and any or all those enticing numbers may have changed.

181

LOW-CARBOHYDRATE DOESN'T ALWAYS MEAN "GOOD FOR YOU" ■ Read package labels carefully. Many times a food or snack will contain a small quantity of carbohydrates—but it will be high in calories because it is high in fat. And somewhere on the label in microscopic print will appear the words: "Not a low-calorie food."

Similarly, a food will claim low calories, carbohydrates, and fat—but for an unrealistically tiny portion. If you suspect this mendacious tactic, double the calories and other numbers for a realistic portion size, and then see if it *still* looks like a dieter's dream.

182 **PEEL APPEAL** ■ Don't peel apples or pears before you eat them. The peels contain most of the fiber, nutrients, and antioxidants that are so vital to our health. Wash the fruits first to get rid of any pesticides.

183 **SPY A DELICIOUS WAY TO KEEP THE DOCTOR AWAY** ■ The variety of apples you eat makes a big difference, with Red Delicious and Northern Spy topping the list of highest oxidant levels. In a Canadian study of eight apple varieties, antioxidant levels were five times higher in the skin of Red Delicious than in its flesh, and three times higher in the skin of Northern Spy than in its flesh. Empire was at the bottom of the barrel, with less than half the antioxidant concentration of Red Delicious.

184 **DELICIOUS FIBER FOODS** ■ Tasty fiber is not an oxymoron. We don't have to eat stuff that tastes like sawdust or drink gritty supplements to get the 20 to 35 grams of fiber per day that doctors recommend.

Here are some tempting choices:

	GRAMS OF FIBER PER SERVING
Legumes	
Pinto beans (½ cup)	10
Red kidney beans (½ cup)	8
Black beans (½ cup)	7
Grains	
Buckwheat groats (kasha) (½ cup)	10
Barley (½ cup)	7
Fruits	
Raspberries	8
Blackberries	7

	GRAMS OF FIBER PER SERVING
Apple	6
Mango	4
Vegetables	
Avocado	9
Acorn squash	9
Artichoke	6
Sweet potato	5

The numbers really tail off from here. If you don't see your favorite food, it wasn't in the top three or four in its category for fiber content.

185 **TINY TREATS HEAD OFF DIET DISASTERS** ■ Sometimes you get the urge for a snack or candy that can contain several hundred calories and lots of carbohydrates and fat. Try a sugar-free, fat-free treat *with the same flavor* instead. For example, instead of a chocolate peanut-butter cup, or even a serving of peanut butter, try a little treat that promises only 4 calories in a two-piece package. The package weighs only 2.2 grams and is clearly labeled "Not a low calorie food." But the flavor of these tiny treats is so intense that it may satisfy your urge.

186 **SUGAR ALCOHOLS CAN CAUSE GASTROINTESTINAL WOES** ■ Sugar alcohols are used as sweeteners in "sugar-free" foods. Look for ingredients that end in "itol" to identify them. Mannitol, sorbitol, and xylitol are the most common, erithritol, lactilol, and maltilol are also used. If you are sensitive to sugar alcohols, as little as 10 to 15 grams—the amount in one serving of sweetened food—can trigger severe gastrointestinal pain and problems.

187 **MAKE SUPERMARKET DESIGN WORK FOR YOU** ■ Most supermarkets share a similar layout, with refrigerated cases along the outside walls. These contain dairy, meat, fish, and frozen foods. Produce is usually located on an unrefrigerated outside wall, and packaged foods and nonfood items are placed on shelves in the middle of the store.

People who want to eat healthfully should choose most of their foods from the fresh or frozen areas. Shopping from these outside aisles also saves lots of time.

188 **NEVER SHOP ON AN EMPTY STOMACH** ■ When you are hungry, you are much more likely to buy food on impulse, and that usually means snack foods. Grab some cubes of low-fat cheese, some slices of turkey breast, or a piece of fruit as you head out the door, and you won't be tempted. Your food bills will be smaller, too.

189 **OUTSMART MINDLESS MUNCHING** ■ If the package of pretzels that was supposed to last all week is gone in an afternoon, you may be a mindless muncher.

You can break this habit, which will help you lose weight.

Keep a food diary and write down all your snacks for one week. Spot your patterns. If you find yourself snacking in the late afternoon, for example, substitute low-fat cheese or a handful of almonds. Take a short break, get out into the fresh air and walk around the block, or phone a friend.

190 **BANISH YOUR GUILT FEELINGS** ■ The binge-and-guilt pattern is very self-destructive and usually leads to more feelings of guilt and more bingeing to feel better.

You'll do better—and lose more weight—if you substitute deep breathing for emotional eating. Deep breathing lowers levels of the stress hormone cortisol, so you're not tempted to soothe yourself with food. Deep breathing also raises levels of serotonin twice as long as any comfort food like pasta.

191

SOME CEREALS AREN'T "BERRY" GOOD FOR YOU ■ Freeze-dried berries or fruit in the new cereals sound like a good thing, but convenience is about all they offer. They contain only a tablespoon or so of the freeze-dried fruit but, thanks to USDA verbiage, it can qualify as a "serving" because this tiny amount will be "reconstituted" with the milk you add to your cereal.

The fruit versions also contain substantially more sugar and less protein and fiber. For example, Cheerios contain 22 grams of carbohydrate, but only 1 gram of sugar and three grams each of protein and fiber. But Apple Cinnamon Cheerios contain 25 grams of carbohydrate, *13 grams of sugar*, 2 grams of protein, and 1 gram of fiber. Strawberry Berry Burst Cheerios contain 24 grams of carbohydrate, *11 grams of sugar*, 3 grams of protein, and 2 grams of fiber. Probably the worst offender is Blueberry Morning, with a whopping 48 grams of carbohydrate, 15 grams of sugar, 4 grams of protein, and 2 grams of fiber.

You'll do much better putting the fruit in yourself. Top high-fiber bran cereal with a sliced apple and a sprinkle of cinnamon, or fresh or freeze-dried berries.

192

GO WILD . . . RICE ■ Switching from white or brown rice to wild rice is a healthy move—and with good reason. Wild rice isn't a member of the rice family, it's an aquatic grass. It has a similar calorie count, but has twice the protein, fiber, and potassium, almost four times as much potassium, six times the iron, seven times the vitamin B_1, twenty-four times the vitamin B_2, and almost four times the vitamin B_3 as white rice.

Although wild rice looks expensive, it quadruples when cooked, so an 8-ounce package makes 6–8 servings.

193

AVOID TRANS FATS ■ Trans-fatty acids ("trans fats" for short) can raise cholesterol and promote heart disease. They are even worse than saturated fats. In 2006, trans-fatty acids must be identified in food labels, and many companies are already removing these dangerous fats from their snacks and are announcing the change on the packages.

Until the new labeling becomes law, the words "hydrogenated" and "partially hydrogenated" will identify trans-fat content.

194

KEEP YOUR LIQUIDS NO-CALORIE OR LOW-CALORIE ■ Unfortunately, our brains don't register the calories in liquids. That's because they don't stay in our stomachs long enough for us to begin to feel full. As a result, many thoughtful nutritionists call soda "liquid candy" and criticize the supersizing of servings from 12 ounces, with 150 calories, 44 grams of carbohydrate, and the equivalent of 10 teaspoons of sugar some years ago to the current 20 ounces, with 250 calories, 65 grams of carbohydrates, and the equivalent of 17 teaspoons of sugar. The 7-Eleven Double Gulp is the prizewinner, with over 600 calories, over 200 grams of carbohydrate, and the equivalent of 52 teaspoons of sugar.

Diet soda is an obvious solution to this sugary problem, but flavored seltzer, with 0 calories and 0 grams of carbohydrate per serving may be a healthier alternative, as it contains no artificial coloring.

195

DON'T BUY FOOD FOR "COMPANY" UNTIL THE DAY THEY'RE EXPECTED ■ We've all made this mistake: We buy special food because we're expecting guests, and we've been trained to be hospitable. That means offering them food.

But these treats are tempting, and often we succumb and start snacking on them. To avoid temptation *and* weight gain *and* sabotaging your blood glucose, delay buying goodies for your guests until the last minute.

196

PRAY YOUR WEIGHT OFF ■ Prayer is said to move mountains, and recent research shows that it can also melt mountains of flesh.

Supporters claim that prayer or meditation soothes your brain's stress center so that it does not produce cortisol. Cortisol is a hormone that makes your heart race and increases your appetite for fatty food. Instead, your brain produces serotonin, the hormone that makes you feel happy, relaxed, and not hungry—especially for high-calorie carbohydrates. As a result, you'll lose weight more easily because you are not eating out of anxiety or stress.

Advocates of this plan urge you to pray or meditate before each meal and whenever your resolve starts wobbling, and to write your prayer, which can be customized for boredom or emotional eaters, on index cards that you can put on the refrigerator, in your wallet, or on your desk.

197 CHOOSE SAFER SNACKS ■ Have veggies dipped in salsa, not chips dunked in dip. (Veggies also take longer to eat.).

Turkey has less than half the calories and only a fraction of the fat of prime rib.

No surprise here: Fresh fruits and berries are more healthful than buffalo wings. Even pretzels are.

198 GO FOR SINGLE SERVINGS ■ Savvy consumers can be blindsided by choosing the "giant economy size" of a treat because it has the lowest cost per serving. But this is *not* a good deal for dieters.

Buy the more expensive single serving of a snack to avoid pigging out. This way you won't be able to overeat.

199 BUFFETS CAN TORPEDO YOUR DIET . . . ■ People respond to variety, and that's the problem with buffets. "All you can eat"—and so many choices!

Scientists actually discovered that people consumed more calories when they were given three different *colors* of pasta, even though they were identical. When the scientists repeated the experiment with three different *shapes* of the same pasta, the results were the same: Their subjects ate more again.

Here's the solution: Take tiny portions of the most interesting-looking foods. Taste them, and then go back to the buffet only once for the two or three dishes that you liked best.

200 **... AND SO CAN DRINKING** ■ Drinking affects your weight in two major ways. Not only does it add calories and carbohydrates to your diet, but it also lowers your inhibitions and resolve not to overeat.

Do some damage control. Don't drink on an empty stomach. Nurse your drinks. Drink wine spritzers—heavy on the club soda, please—or alcoholic drinks that use lots of diet soda or tonic.

201 **AN APPETIZING STRATEGY** ■ Order two appetizers instead of a main course. You'll actually eat less.

202 **JOIN A SUPPORT GROUP** ■ The success of support groups like Weight Watchers and Overeaters Anonymous is well known. Some newer support groups, which may be even more useful, are specifically for people with diabetes. (Being an admittedly impatient New Yorker, I'd try a support for three meetings, then decide whether it's worth continuing to go.)

203 **KNOW WHERE DANGEROUS TRANS FATS LURK** ■ Trans fats (partially hydrogenated oils) have been linked to coronary disease and strokes. Knowing which types of foods are most likely to contain trans fats will help you avoid buying and eating them. Among the culprits:

Cakes
Cookies
Crackers
Doughnuts

Foods fried in (partially) hydrogenated fats—e.g., chicken, fish,
  potatoes
Margarines (some)
Pies
Vegetable shortenings

204 AVOID "DIET" BARS AND SHAKES ■ "Diet" bars and shakes are loaded with many kinds of sugar. Some of the bars contain as many as 30–35 grams of carbohydrates and an entire thesaurus of sugars. Some bars contain as many as *eight* different kinds of sugar: corn syrup, high-fructose corn syrup, sugar, brown sugar, maltodextrin, dextrose, honey, and high-maltose corn syrup. (And also trans fats!)

The first seven ingredients of one diet shake are fructose (sugar), maltodextrin (sugar), cocoa, dextrose (sugar), soy protein, sugar, and cornstarch (rapidly metabolized into sugar).

205 BECOME A "SWEETS SNOB" ■ Make the bargain with yourself—and keep it!—to pass up trash-food carbs and indulge only in gourmet goodies. You can quash a craving better with *one* chocolatier's truffle than with a mass-produced mostly corn syrup candy bar from the vending machine, or a whole bag of bargain chocolate-chip cookies—and you'd come out ahead calorie- and sugarwise. Training yourself to savor one high-class treat is cheaper, smarter, and better for your body *and* your self-esteem!

206 PUT A FACE ON YOUR SLIPS AND CHOICES ■ The sneakiest part of diabetes is that you don't pay for today's binge until sometime down the road instead of paying the price immediately. Sit down and examine some real equivalents: Today's candy bar could take one day off your vision in ten years; the sour cream and butter and carbs in today's loaded baked potato could be worth two toes in three birthdays. Having a clear picture of what an indulgence costs really helps you say no without feeling martyred because you know what you're trading for with your choice.

207 **DEFAT BEFORE DIGGING IN** ■ Cut the fat from your soups and stews, and you'll cut calories without sacrificing the taste. Just toss three or four ice cubes into the pot, or one into each bowl. Wait one minute, then scoop out the ice and the congealed fat, and discard them.

(If you are cooking today for tomorrow's dinner, refrigerating the dish for at least four hours will solidify all the fat, which you can then remove easily.)

208 **EXPERIMENT WITH MARINADES** ■ Brushing meat or fish with marinade can completely change its flavor. (For me, it's probably the only way I'll eat chicken breast three times a week.)

Start with a liquid—vegetable juice (lemon, tomato, or vegetable other than carrot) or flavored vinegar (balsamic, sherry, red or white wine), and add herbs and spices (freeze-dried onion, shallots, or garlic, a mix of peppers, chives, rosemary, basil, tarragon, or a premixed blend, like McCormick's).

Take notes so you'll remember your successes.

209 **RECOGNIZE THAT SUGAR IS AN ADDICTION** ■ Many recent research studies have linked sugar consumption to major medical problems, not the least of which is the present epidemic of obesity in the industrialized world. In the United States alone, our rate is now 158 pounds of sugar per year for every man, woman, and child—*almost one-half pound every single day.*

Possibly the best book on the subject was published back in 1975: *Sugar Blues* by William Dufty, which connects refined sugar to a laundry list of diseases in coruscating detail and proves his case through the centuries, with many historical documents.

The best way to determine whether sugar is an addiction for *you* is to examine your own eating patterns. If you find that these tempting white crystals are as addictive as narcotics and are turning you into a "sugar junkie," go cold turkey as though sugar were a hard drug. Your diabetes will improve dramatically.

210 **BROWN SUGAR AND HONEY AREN'T MUCH BETTER** ■ Sure, brown sugar is less refined than white, and honey is a natural food that fearless cavemen fought bees and bears to feast on. However, practically speaking, while honey contains antioxidants and many B vitamins, it cannot be considered a significant source of them. About the only benefit of honey is that there are hundreds of varieties, and that the rich subtlety of its taste may limit the size of your serving.

211 **DON'T LET THE POUNDS CREEP UP** ■ It's a sad fact of life that the average adult gains two pounds per year just because of slowing metabolism. Doesn't sound like much, but it translates to twenty pounds per decade.

Keep an eye on the scale and try to be more active—even if it's just a short walk after dinner.

It's easier to lose five pounds than fifty!

212 **IT'S GREAT TO GRATE** ■ Add lots of powerful flavor with no or minimal calories by grating small quantities of savory foods on top of your dishes.

Try hard cheeses, nuts, nutmeg, orange, lemon, and lime rinds.

213 **SHAPE CONTROLS CONSUMPTION** ■ We oughtta be smarter and not influenced by optical illusions. Nevertheless, people pour more liquid into—and then drink more out of—short, wide glasses than tall, narrow ones holding the same number of ounces.

Choose the long, skinny glass every time!

214 **RESTAURANT SAVVY VI: BE PROUD YOU'RE PARTICULAR** ■ There's no need to flinch over asking a waiter what's in a dish, or can the cream be left out, or how many ounces in a portion. If he doesn't know—and really, he should—he can ask the kitchen. We live in a world of lactose-intolerant people, wheat-sensitive people, Atkins and Zone Diet adherents, and all sorts of other eating problems and programs. As long as you are polite, reasonable, and specific in your request, don't shy away from asking for some special adjustment. And if the waiter is gracious and compliant, please tip a little extra!

215 **RESTAURANT SAVVY VII: DON'T LET A MENU BLOW YOUR FUSES** ■ Too many restaurant menus have too many choices—and too many temptations. Sometimes reading florid descriptions of dishes is all it takes to kick up a craving, so don't. Rather than let the options lead you, see what you're in the mood for and choose without even opening the menu. That way, you will order exactly what you want—or something very much like it—without being seduced by what the restaurant wants to sell you.

216 **RESTAURANT SAVVY VIII: WHY REINVENT THE WHEEL WHEN SOMEONE'S ALREADY DONE IT FOR YOU?** ■ The key to eating food prepared by others is knowing what you're eating, and how much you're consuming. Many chain restaurants regulate their recipes and portion sizes, and have that information available on request; choose those establishments. Check the menu for nutrition information, or ask your server whether pamphlets with those details are available.

217 **RESTAURANT SAVVY IX: "SUPERSIZE" IS A FOUR-LETTER WORD** ■ Extra-hearty portions mean extra calories, extra exchanges, and extra trouble on a platter. If you suspect that a serving will be bigger than it should be, don't even let it hit your plate. Ask the kitchen to serve you only *half* of their customary portion, and to wrap the rest "to go." Clever you—you'll treat your taste buds to what they really wanted, feel no deprivation because you've finished everything on your plate, and even carry away tomorrow's lunch or dinner!

218 **RESTAURANT SAVVY X: BUFFET SUCCESS ▪** Buffets are only for the truly disciplined. The good news is that you can sample a bit of this and a taste of that, and have a great time grazing. The horrible news is that the entire array is laid out to tempt you, with heavy-mayonnaise-and-pasta dishes right next to the carrot sticks. Even worse, there's no portion control; you have no idea how much you're taking in. If you're part of a group determined to gorge at a smorgasbord, you can go along—just don't even look at the layout. Specify your needs, and ask a trusted friend to fill a plate for you. *Just one.*

219 **RESTAURANT SAVVY XI: NEVER EAT WHAT YOU DON'T RECOGNIZE ▪** Stay with food you recognize and know how to count: a small baked white or sweet potato, green vegetables, grilled skinless chicken breasts or fish, steaks listed as "six ounces," etc. Avoid dishes that combine several foods in unknown amounts because you can't even guess well—or count exchanges. Something baked, grilled, broiled, or poached is always preferable to something fried, sautéed, or breaded. And if your entree comes covered with gravy or sauce, send it back and ask for the same thing, but "naked."

220 **THE DEVIL'S IN THE DENSITY ▪** Suppose you knew that a 3- or 4-ounce portion of a food contained 1,000 calories. (Many fast foods do.) Wouldn't eating it frequently make you put on weight?

A high number of calories per ounce of food is called "energy (calorie) density." Unfortunately, the appetite-control center in your brain signals feelings of fullness after a certain *weight* or *volume* of food has been eaten, rather than a certain number of calories.

And that's why you'll never put on weight gorging on celery sticks!

(For more information, read "Fast foods, energy density and obesity: a possible mechanistic link" by A. M. Prentice and S. A. Jebb in the November 2003 issue of *Obesity Reviews,* available on the Internet.)

221

NO CATCH IN THIS RYE ■ Eating rye bread causes a smaller insulin response than does wheat bread. Researchers tested types of rye bread, containing different amounts of fiber, but concluded that the lower response was not due to the fiber content, which varied. Experiments showed that rye starch metabolized more slowly than did wheat starch.

222

BE SKEPTICAL OF THE DIETARY GUIDELINES ADVISORY COMMITTEE ■ We'd all like to believe that the members of the Dietary Guidelines Advisory Committee, a group that reviews scientific papers on health and nutrition and advises the U.S. Department of Health & Human Services and the Department of Agriculture on revisions to Americans' dietary guidelines, are impartial and unbiased.

We'd be very naïve. According to the watchdog group Center for Science in the Public Interest, some DGAC members have received substantial funding from the sugar, dairy, and other food-industry groups and drug companies. Two members in particular have close ties and possible conflicts of interest. One, who has conducted research funded by the Sugar Association, has urged the U.S. Food & Drug Administration not to list refined sugars on food labels. Another has worked closely with the American Council on Science & Health, an industry group that minimizes virtually every food-related health concern, including trans fats.

Bottom line: Find trustworthy independent verification of any DGAC report, or ignore it. You can guess who's buttering their bread!

223 DEFEAT DIET SABOTEURS I: "I MADE YOUR FAVORITE DISH" ■ Loving partners, mothers, grandmothers, siblings, aunts, and children can be the most powerful diet saboteurs because they know how to push our buttons and make us feel guilty for refusing them.

Here are two simple strategies to defeat them: Say "Darling, I'll have just a forkful—or spoonful," and stick to your guns, or "Darling, you'll have to phone my doctor for permission. Here's the phone number."

224 DEFEAT DIET SABOTEURS II: FRIENDS AND COWORKERS ■ Sometimes these folks are well-meaning; sometimes they have hidden agendas, like the friends who don't want you to succeed at losing weight because they need to lose weight, too.

Again, here are two simple strategies for outwitting them: Play with the food on your plate, but don't eat it or eat only a tiny bit. Hope that osmosis will make the food melt into your plate. Or say simply, "I'd love to try this, but my allergies would make me break out in hives." You'll be off the hook!

225 THE *REAL* SEAFOOD DIET ■ You know the old joke: "I'm on a seafood diet. I seafood, I eat it."

But a seafood diet is extremely low in calories and can help you lose weight. A 6-ounce serving of fish or shellfish contains less than 250 calories, with virtually no fat. In contrast, a 6-ounce serving of lean broiled beef can contain 450–500 calories, with 20–30 grams of fat. Pork has even more calories and is even higher in fat. Lamb, veal, and chicken are better, but are still much higher than seafood.

226 THE LURE OF LOBSTER ■ Lobster is the best "diet bar-gain." A 7-ounce portion of lobster meat (equal to a one-pound lobster) contains less than 200 calories and 2 grams of fat, and provides a whopping 35 grams of protein.

Eating a steamed or broiled lobster is time-consuming, so you'll definitely feel full. It is "fiddle food" par excellence!

Note: Most Northeastern cities have stores where you can buy live lobsters wholesale. Culls—lobsters that have lost one claw in a fight—are special bargains!

227 THE SWEET ADDICTION ■ Eating sweets can trigger the desire to eat more and more of them. Curb your craving by delaying these delights until *after* you eat a meal or snack that contains protein. You'll be less likely to go overboard.

228 CHART YOUR WEIGHT LOSS ■ A column of numbers showing your weekly weight may be OK, but you'll become more motivated by seeing a downward-sloping line on a chart. Post it on your refrigerator, where it will act as a continuing inspiration.

229 KNOW THE DIFFERENCE BETWEEN YOUR NATURAL WEIGHT AND YOUR IDEALIZED WEIGHT ■ Your idealized weight is a product of insurance-company statistics. It is formulaic and represents hundreds of thousands of people. For many of us, it has little connection to reality.

Instead, strive for your "natural weight"—what you weighed when you were in your twenties, if you were somewhat active. Chances are that you will never have the shape of a *Vogue* or *GQ* model, but they have to starve themselves because the camera makes them appear twenty pounds heavier. Ditch any unrealistic weight-loss expectations, but keep focused on achievable goals.

230 CALCIUM MAY BOOST WEIGHT LOSS ■ According to one study, Americans who consume the lowest average level of calcium (255 milligrams per day) are 84 percent more likely to be overweight than those consuming that highest average level (1,364 milligrams per day).

Low-calcium diets make the body release calcitriol, a hormone that not only increases absorption of calcium in the intestines, so that you get the most calcium possible from food, but also makes your fat cells make and store more fat.

Note: The calcium from dairy foods was more effective than calcium supplements, perhaps owing to the nutrients in the food.

231 **MAKE PEACE WITH FOOD ■** Food is not your friend. Food is not your enemy. Food is simply food—nourishment—and sometimes it's delicious.

It's time to "decriminalize" food and to savor the best of it. *Slowly.*

232 **ORANGE YOU SMART I: AN ORANGE A DAY ■** Oranges may do more for your health than the proverbial daily apple. The citrus fruits can help prevent certain oral and gastrointestinal cancers, according to a new Australian study. The study also found "convincing evidence" that citrus fruits could reduce risk of obesity, diabetes, and cardiovascular diseases.

Oranges possess the highest level of antioxidants of all fruits, with more than 170 different phytochemicals, including over 60 bioflavonoids having anti-inflammatory and antitumor properties.

233 **ORANGE YOU SMART II: EAT MORE ORANGE FOODS ■** Orange-colored foods are extremely high in antioxidants, phytochemicals, and bioflavonoids, but are not always inexpensive or easy to find, especially during the winter. Look for dried apricots (but don't eat too many at one time), sweet potatoes, winter squash, and, when you can find them, orange sweet peppers imported from Holland. (Eat carrots, too, if they don't raise your blood glucose too much.)

234 **GET NUTTY II ■** Nuts are an excellent source of protein, minerals like manganese and zinc, and B vitamins and folate. Walnuts, almonds, and pecans are especially rich in these nutrients, although the calorie counts and nutritional content vary slightly.

Note: Peanuts and coconut belong to other botanical classes. Peanuts are legumes, like beans and peas, but are eaten like other nuts and are closer to nuts than to beans in their nutritional composition. The coconut is a drupe—a fruit with a hard pit, like a cherry or plum.

Warning: Coconut is even higher in saturated fats and calories than red meat is. If you adore coconut, use it very sparingly as a garnish.

235 **HEALTHY DESSERT ■** I owe this quick, easy treat to my late grandmother, who always served this to guests, with or without dinner. Just stuff dried apricots or pitted prunes with walnut halves and serve them in a pretty crystal dish. (My grandmother rolled these morsels in sugar, but we know better, and they are tastier without all the additional sweetening.) One caution: Because pieces of fruit or nuts look so small, they may seem harmless, but in fact they're concentrated sugar—so limit yourself to just a few pieces a day.

236 **SNACK ON SUNFLOWER SEEDS ■** Sunflower seeds are high in fiber, vitamin E, calcium, protein, and polyunsaturated fat, and low in carbohydrates and sugars. Grow the tall, beautiful flowers in your yard or on your terrace and pull out the ripe seeds, or buy the unsalted variety in a health-food store. Sunflower seeds—and the equally tasty pumpkin seeds—have been harvested and used by Native Americans for thousands of years, even ground into flour.

Additional snacking bonus: Cracking the seeds in your teeth slows down your rate of consumption.

237 **FLAVORED COFFEE FOR DESSERT ■** Save hundreds of calories by choosing a flavored coffee for dessert. Opt for gourmet varieties like hazelnut, chocolate raspberry, mocha, or vanilla. All of them have so few calories that you can even top your coffee with *one* teaspoon of ice cream and still stay under 50 calories.

238 GOURMET TEAS FOR HEALTH ■ Green, black, and herbal teas are all rich in flavonoids, which provide cardiovascular benefits. Recent research indicates that frequent tea drinking may affect the endothelium (the lining of the heart) favorably, which can help protect your heart from cardiovascular disease.

239 BET ON BERRIES ■ All fresh berries are marvelous nutritional bargains. One delicious filling cup of berries will cost you anywhere from 45 calories and 10 grams of carbohydrate for strawberries up to only 82 calories and 20 grams of carbohydrate for blueberries. Raspberries and blackberries fall in between. In addition, they are loaded with antioxidants and phytochemicals.

Frozen whole berries offer essentially the same nutrients as fresh berries, but have a mushy texture so they work better as ingredients in a dish, rather than being eaten alone. Just make sure that they have been frozen without sugar!

240 AN OUNCE OF PREVENTION IS WORTH POINTS ON YOUR GLUCOMETER ■ Many diabetics use those "I need something right now" moments to justify grabbing some snack they shouldn't. Plan ahead to outwit those occasions. Keep cut-up veggies in plastic containers in the refrigerator, or in plastic bags in your briefcase. Carry one-ounce portions of peanuts, almonds, or walnuts in your purse or pocket. Make those "grab something" moments into "grab something *smart*" moments and do yourself a favor instead of an injury.

241 SNACK WELL ON POPCORN ■ Popcorn is a healthy nibble *if* you make it yourself—and it's much fresher tasting, too. Most "manufactured" popcorn was packaged months ago, and made with trans fats.

Packaged microwave popcorn is fresher, but not necessarily better nutritionally, as it often contains trans fats, too.

But *you* can make your popcorn from scratch in your microwave; the hot air will make it pop without any oil. When you make popcorn this way, it's a dieter's dream. Three tablespoons of unpopped kernels will produce one serving of 6 cups popped, which contains 110 calories, 27 grams of carbohydrate, only 1 gram of sugar, 4 grams of protein, and a hefty 7 grams of fiber.

Buying popcorn in the kernel is a bargain hunter's dream, too. You can usually find a two-pound bag, which will produce twenty-three servings, in your supermarket for around $2.

242 **PUT PARSLEY ON EVERYTHING** ■ Parsley is a dieter's friend. An entire cup contains only 22 calories, with 4 grams of carbohydrate, 1 gram of sugar, 2 grams of fiber, and 2 grams of protein. It provides 101 percent of the Recommended Daily Allowance of vitamin A, 133 percent of the RDA of vitamin C, and is a very good source of calcium, copper, folate, iron, magnesium, and potassium.

So make parsley part of your cuisine. Put it into soups, stews, and salads, use it as a garnish, and nibble it all by itself.

243 **WEIGHT LOSS REDUCES ARTHRITIS RISK** ■ If you are ten to twenty pounds overweight, losing as little as ten of those excess pounds will reduce your risk of developing osteoarthritis by 50 percent, according to John Klippel, M.D., president and CEO of the Arthritis Foundation.

If you are more than twenty pounds overweight, you will need to lose more than ten pounds to reduce your osteoarthritis risk significantly. It's definitely worth it!

244 **TRY THE "WHITE-OUT" DIET** ■ Many diabetics can achieve substantial weight loss with a "white-out" diet: eliminating white bread, flour, rice, sugar (in its many forms), and potatoes. No surprise—all of these foods have high glycemic indexes and make most diabetics' blood glucose rise quickly.

245 **SUBSTITUTE CAROB FOR COCOA?** ■ Health-food fans support the strategy; chocoholics think it's heresy.

The answer probably lies somewhere in between. Compared to cocoa, carob powder—sometimes called "carob flour"—is only slightly lower in calories, but contains more than twice as many grains of carbohydrate, half of which are sugar. Carob contains three times as much fiber, but no protein or iron, and cocoa contains both. Carob has no fat, but cocoa contains very little.

Before artificial sweeteners were available, the natural sweetness of carob was an advantage because its users did not have to add sugar the way cocoa users did. And the sugar added all the calories and carbohydrates.

Now the playing field is more level. Chocolate lovers can choose based on their taste preferences.

246 **RECOMMENDED NUTRITION WEB SITE** ■ We diabetics quickly become amateur nutritionists—we have to be. This wonderful Web site makes it easy and fun to choose foods that are good for us: www.nutritiondata.com.

When you log on and type in the food you are looking for, you will find a four-page printout that is a biochemist's delight.

But let's take it from the top. After you type in the food, which can include branded or processed foods, you will see a box that contains basic nutrition facts, based on U.S. Department of Agriculture analysis: serving size, calories, calories from fat, total carbohydrates, sugars, protein, and several vitamins and minerals.

A brightly colored pyramid shows you the food's composition in percentages (carbohydrates, fats, and protein), rates the food on a five-star scale, and lists what's good and what's bad about the food. (Remember: the problem with nutrition sites that rate foods is that they often rate them based on how closely they come to the Food Pyramid, which not everyone agrees is a healthy diet.)

Serious students of nutrition can then see a three-page nutritional analysis of the food: all the different "oses" that make up the sugar content, all the different proteins and amino acids, the vitamins, minerals, and bar charts illustrating whether the food scores high or low on each element per 200 calories.

This is a fascinating Web site that will help you make more intelligent choices about what you eat.

247 THE "SKINNY" ON FAST FOODS ■ Look at www.nutritiondata.com for a comprehensive analysis of fast foods, too.

Although the Web site listed only eighteen restaurant chains as of January 2004, there are as many as eighty-six different menu items per chain.

248 COCKTAIL PARTY STRATEGY ■ Ya gotta walk around with a drink in your hand, right? But that means you can't hold an hors d'oeuvre in that hand!

Here are some look-alike drinks that will keep your calories and alcohol consumption down:

Virgin Mary instead of a Bloody Mary
Club soda or tonic with a wedge of lime instead of gin (or vodka)
    and tonic
Or substitute a wine spritzer for a glass of wine

249 RESIST NIBBLING WITH REST ■ Dieters who get enough sleep find it easier to stay with their weight-loss programs. According to recent research, dieters who classified themselves as "well-rested," snacked less and lost more weight than those who said they weren't getting enough sleep.

Try a catnap instead of cookies to restore your energy!

250 THE ORAC DIMENSION ■ You already know that you should be consuming lots of antioxidants to keep healthy and prevent damage by free radicals. A new table that lists foods scoring high in an antioxidant assay called ORAC (Oxygen Radical Absorbance Capacity) is extremely valuable. The survey recommends consuming at least 3,000 ORAC units a day and lists top antioxidant foods by ORAC units per 100 grams (approximately 3½ ounces).

Fruits run far ahead of vegetables in this ranking. Prunes lead the list with 5,770 units, which means that 50 grams (less than 2 ounces) would meet the requirement. Raisins are in second place with 2,830 ORAC units, followed by blueberries (2,400) and blackberries (2,036). Strawberries and raspberries rank much lower.

Kale is the highest-ranking vegetable, with 1,770 units, followed by spinach, with 1,260.

251 LOW-CARBOHYDRATE DIET? CONSULT YOUR DOCTOR AND LOWER YOUR INSULIN ■
It's not because your doctor will try to persuade you to choose a "more balanced" diet. In fact, many doctors have lost weight on Atkins and other low-carbohydrate diets and are among their most vocal supporters.

But if your insulin and other hypoglycemic drugs are not lowered, you can go into sudden shock and die. Case in point, told to me by a prominent Manhattan internist who is a happy Atkins dieter:

One of his patients, a diabetic in his thirties, went on the Atkins diet without having his insulin dosage changed—and died quite suddenly from hypoglycemic shock.

So—to reiterate—*if you are lowering your carbohydrate intake, you must have your insulin and other hypoglycemic drugs lowered.*

252 DON'T DRINK TOO MUCH WATER AT ONE TIME ■
Drinking too much water at one time is dangerous. It's very tempting to drink a quart of water or more within a few minutes to make sure you get your daily quota, but drinking too much water too quickly leads to a dangerous dilution of the salt and other electrolytes in your blood, causing "water intoxication" that may require hospitalization. Older people are especially vulnerable to this serious problem.

Instead, unless you have been exercising or it is very hot, drink only a cup or two of water at a time. Let your thirst be your guide.

253 **BETCHA *CAN* EAT JUST ONE** ■ Many calorie, carbohydrate, and fat counts for snacks are based on a serving of more than one piece. A serving of Hershey Kisses, for example, is based on nine pieces and contains 230 calories, 24 grams of carbohydrate, and 13 grams of fat.

Try eating just one, letting it dissolve slowly and pleasurably in your mouth. Then you're talking about a very manageable 25 calories, 2.7 grams of carbohydrate, and 1.5 grams of fat.

254 **TRY SIX LITTLE MEALS A DAY** ■ You may be able to lose more weight on six little meals a day. Same number of daily calories, if you're counting them, but spread out more.

Such a weight-loss program works for many dieters—not just diabetics—for two major reasons: (1) They are less tempted to overeat because they are eating so often, and (2) the frequent meals keep their metabolic furnace stoked up, so they burn more calories.

255 **OLESTRA WOES** ■ Olestra (trademarked Olean)—the indigestible "fat-free" fat substitute—can cause gastrointestinal havoc. Some people suffer such severe diarrhea or cramps that they wind up in the emergency room. Olestra also reduces your body's absorption of carotenoids, which are vital nutrients.

If you get the urge for fat-free potato chips, try Tip No. 73: "Guilt-free Potato Chips."

256 **BUY THE FAMILY SIZE, THEN DIVIDE** ■ Supermarkets often put cuts of meat and fish in "family-size" packages, which can save you over $1 per pound.

Take advantage of these bargains, then cut and wrap individual portions and freeze them.

257 TRY BROCHETTES ■ Brochettes are a tasty quick-fix dish. You've probably tasted shishkebab, but brochettes come in many varieties, low in calories and fat, high in protein and vitamins.

Thread cubes of meat, chicken, or fish on a skewer, alternating with chunks of onion, pepper, tomato, or other vegetables. Broil in the oven or rotisserie, or on the barbecue.

258 EXPERIMENT WITH STIR-FRIES ■ Stir-fry recipes are another tasty way to increase the vegetable content of your dinners. Try stir-fries with asparagus, snow peas, spinach, Chinese cabbage (bok choy), broccoli, hot or sweet peppers, Chinese mushrooms, or scallions.

259 DROP THE TWO-HOUR LUNCH ■ Two-hour lunches are too tempting. Too many opportunities to eat too much food, or just sit around, which slows your metabolism.

Instead, take only an hour and one-quarter for lunch, then go shopping or take a walk with your lunch companion.

260 AVOID OVERLY RESTRICTIVE DIETS ■ Sure, they may work for a week or two, but they may also create a feeling of deprivation. When it gets too strong, your diet may backfire and cause you to go on an eating jag. It's much smarter to start your diet by making a list of *ten or twelve foods* that you absolutely will not eat. Anything else is OK as long as you control your portions.

261 DON'T QUIT SMOKING AND START DIETING AT THE SAME TIME ■ Taking on two deprivations at once is almost a recipe for failure. Quit smoking first. Not only will it start you on the way to a healthier future, but you will also redeem your taste buds. When you begin your diet a month or two later, you will really savor your food and find it easier to lose weight.

262 SPEND YOUR FAST-FOOD ALLOWANCE ON KITCHEN GADGETS ■ Whether it's a pepper or salt mill, an apple corer, a cherry pitter, a lemon zester, or mushroom slicer, it's an inexpensive investment in making food look and taste better quickly and easily. Doesn't that make more sense than spending your money on fast-food meals or coffee breaks?

263 PICTURE PERFECT ■ Make the old adage, "One picture is worth a thousand words" reinforce your weight-loss plan.

Put some photos on your refrigerator for continuing inspiration. You could choose a photo of yourself when you were in high school or college, or a newlywed, and weighed much less. You could attach your face to a movie star's or athlete's body—preferably in a bathing suit. Write the caption "MY GOAL" on it and keep on focusing on that goal—especially every time you go to the refrigerator.

Note: If negative stimuli inspire you more, put a photo of yourself at your present weight on the fridge.

264 SUPPLEMENT A MICROWAVE MEAL WITH A GREEN SALAD AND FRESH FRUIT ■ Microwave meals can be lifesavers after a long day at work. Make them healthier by adding a green salad and fresh fruit or berries for more fiber, vitamins, and antioxidants.

265 STAY AWAY FROM CEREAL BARS ■ Cereal bars are a poor nutritional bargain. They are promoted as a quick, portable breakfast, but many of them are loaded with all kinds of sugars and trans fats. (What really irks me is seeing "high fructose corn syrup" first or second on the listed of ingredients, followed immediately by "corn syrup." Now, really!!!)

Some cereal bars are somewhat more nutritious. Look for labeling that says "no hydrogenated oils." They are certainly better for you than a bagel, muffin, or doughnut!

266 PUT YOUR PET ON A DIET, TOO ■ Many dogs and cats are now as overweight or obese as their loving owners. As a result, many of them have become diabetic, with all the cardiovascular risk that their owners face.

The best thing you can do to increase your pet's life—and your own—is put both of you on a diet. Limit snacks and increase exercise. Check first with your vet.

267 BEAN BENEFITS ■ Beans have a lot going for them. Not only are they an excellent source of low-fat protein and fiber, but they also provide substantial iron and folic acid.

I like the versatility of beans—especially red kidney beans, white beans (cannellini), and pinto beans. With a blender or food processor, you can make a soup or dip very quickly. Or make a bean salad for a nourishing hot-weather dinner.

Recent research suggests that high-fiber beans can increase weight loss by 66 percent, according to a study published in *Nutrition Reviews*. Says Michigan State University nutrition professor Maurice Bennink, Ph.D., "Getting at least 30 grams of fiber a day ($\frac{1}{2}$ cup of kidney beans contains 23 grains) can significantly speed dieting success—even without exercise or other lifestyle changes."

268 CHOCOLATE LOVER? THE DARKER, THE BETTER FOR YOU ■ The most healthful chocolate you can eat is the darkest. Search for chocolate labeled "70 percent cocoa solids," which has the highest concentration of heart-healthy phytochemicals and iron, and very little sugar and carbohydrates.

You can sometimes find pound-plus bars of this gourmet chocolate at specialty supermarkets like Trader Joe's for as little as $3.

269 **YO-YO DIETING INCREASES HEALTH RISKS** ■ Losing weight and regaining it all, then losing weight again and gaining it back has some harmful consequences. This yo-yo dieting seems to increase the risk of cardiovascular disease, already the number-one killer of women in the United States. Yo-yo dieting can also lower the levels of the "good" HDL cholesterol and raise triglycerides, an independent risk factor for heart disease in women.

270 **TRY THE TRIPLE-MIRROR TEST** ■ Sometime during the winter holidays, you may need encouragement to stay with your weight-loss plan. (Admittedly, all those parties don't help.) Strengthen your resolve by going to an upscale department store that has a cruisewear department and try on some bathing suits in a triple-mirrored dressing room. Look at your body from *all* angles. What you see—and what you'd like to see in a few months—may inspire you to stay on the straight and narrow and not abandon your diet.

271 **GIVE YOURSELF A HAND** ■ Maybe you're tired of weighing your food—I know I am!—or there are situations where you can't. Estimate your portion size by comparing it to your hand:

one thumb = 1 tablespoon, or 1 ounce of cheese
one palm (or a deck of cards) = 3 ounces of meat
one fist = 8 ounces of liquid, or 1 cup of solid food

272 **PUMPKINS: NOT JUST FOR PIE** ■ Pumpkins are a wonderful winter food because they are an excellent source of vitamin A (it's their bright orange color!) and such minerals as potassium and phosphorus.

All this nutrition comes at a low caloric cost. One cup of raw pumpkin cubes contains only 30 calories, with 8 grams of carbohydrate and only a trace of fat. If you love pumpkin pie, put the cubes in a blender or food processor, then simmer them with powdered ginger and nutmeg and a sugar substitute for a sweet treat. Or simmer the pumpkin cubes with dried sage to get the taste of pumpkin ravioli without the calories and carbohydrates.

Tip: Pumpkins go on sale November 1, the day after Halloween.

273 **VIM AND VINEGAR . . .** ■ Vinegars contribute a variety of interesting flavors without adding any calories at all. This category has changed a lot in the past ten years as old supermarket standbys like red, white, and cider vinegars have been joined by balsamic, malt, sherry, tarragon, and raspberry.

Try different varieties on salads, vegetables, meat, and fish. Raspberry vinegar is especially tasty on melons, berries, and fruit.

274 **. . . AND OTHER CONDIMENTS AND SAUCES** ■ Here, too, you can add a lot of flavor without adding calories or carbohydrates. An assortment of condiments can make the blandness of chicken breasts disappear. Drizzle them on cooked vegetables to disguise their taste—maybe you'll eat more of them. Tabasco anyone?

275 **"NATURAL" DOESN'T MEAN "HEALTHFUL"** ■ Packaged-food manufacturers love to make their products sound as if they're good for you. The labeling "naturally sweetened" is one of the most insidious sales and marketing tools because it tempts us to buy something—usually a snack—that is nutritious and "good for us."

I've got news for you: Sugar is a natural sweetener. So is molasses, which is made from sugar cane. So is honey. And so—stretching the point just a bit—is xylitol, a sugar alcohol made from birch bark, which causes horrendous gastric problems in many people in portions as small as 10 mg. (one-third ounce). In fact, if sawdust were sweet, it, too, could be labeled a "natural sweetener." (It comes from trees, doesn't it?) If you think I'm kidding, before the 1980s, sawdust was added to many brands of "diet bread" to increase their fiber content.

276 **NEITHER DOES "ORGANIC"** ■ According to U.S. Department of Agriculture labeling, "organic" has to do with certain prohibitions in the way food is grown. Organic foods cannot be genetically engineered or modified, cannot be fertilized by sewage sludge or irradiated, and cannot be fed animal-slaughter byproducts, antibiotics, or growth hormones.

Clearly, then, organic food may be the choice of food purists, "free-range" fans, opponents of agribusinesses, and chefs.

However, that said, the caloric, carbohydrate, and fat content of many packaged "organic" foods may be so high that people with diabetes should avoid them or eat them very sparingly. "Organic" does not mean "You don't have to read the label."

277 **SNEAKY LABELING: "NO CHOLESTEROL"** ■ And now we come to really sneaky labeling: packaged foods marked "no cholesterol." For too many foods, these words are misleading because, while legally true, the food never did contain cholesterol, which comes from *animal* sources.

For example, a package of potato chips fried in coconut oil, which is high in saturated fats that are very harmful to the cardiovascular system, could legally be labeled "no cholesterol." And so could a loaf of bread made with partially hydrogenated vegetable oil, another cardiovascular villain.

A package of frozen vegetables could also be labeled "no cholesterol." Of course, vegetables do not contain cholesterol, anyway—unless they're in butter or cream sauce.

You'll be healthier if you ignore the "no cholesterol" label and concentrate instead on what the food *does* contain.

278 GET THE GOODS ON GRANOLA ■ Granola conjures up all sorts of warm and fuzzy feelings—kind of like yogurt, sandals, and sunshine.

But granola may not be as healthful as the other three for people with diabetes. Many varieties of granola contain partially hydrogenated vegetable oils, 210 calories in a half-cup serving, with 36 grams of carbohydrate and only 4 grams of fiber and 6 grams of protein. (And who eats only one-half cup, anyway?) In contrast, a half-cup serving of Fiber One cereal, contains only 60 calories, 24 grams of carbohydrate, 14 grams of fiber, and 2 grams of protein.

279 WATCH CALORIES AS WELL AS FIBER CONTENT ■ Cereals can be a good source of desirable fiber; we need 30–40 grams of it per day. But cereals are among the most important packaged foods whose labeling you must read very carefully. Even "bran" and "fiber" cereals may contain too many calories, carbohydrates, and sugars to be good for you, and there is a great deal of variation among the hundreds of different brands of cereals.

For example, Post Raisin Bran contains 190 calories in a one-cup serving, with 46 grams of carbohydrate, 8 grams of fiber, and 4 grams of protein. Post Bran Flakes contains 100 calories in a ¾-cup serving, with 24 grams of carbohydrate, 5 grams of fiber, and 3 grams of protein. Original Shredded Wheat, which you might think would be high in fiber, has only 80 calories per biscuit, but also only 2.5 grams of fiber.

280 MAKE FRIENDS WITH YOUR SUPERMARKET MANAGER ■ Make a point of learning your manager's first name and greeting him whenever you see him. Treating him like a person, rather than a job title, lets you find out useful information, like what will be on sale next week, and lets you ask him for favors, like ordering special foods and merchandise for you.

281

KNOW THE DARK SIDE OF SUPERMARKET DESIGN ■
Have you ever wondered why the dairy case is usually in the back of the supermarket? To make you go through lots of aisles and look at lots and lots of merchandise, before you can get to the quart of milk you came in for. That way, maybe you'll buy some other things as well. Supermarkets want you to fill your shopping cart, not buy just one item.

Similarly, staple items are scattered all over supermarkets so that you have to visit every aisle. That's why most people find it difficult to finish the weekly shopping trip in less than fifteen minutes.

Foods with high markups are usually piled attractively in displays at the end of aisles. That's because it takes you a little longer to make the turn—more time for you to be tempted. Other high-markup items are placed at your eye level, or your child's.

Now that you know the secret, you can avoid a lot of that deliberately engineered temptation. Just stick to your shopping list—except maybe for one treat.

282

OUTWIT THE WINTER WEIGHT-GAIN SYNDROME ■
Genetically, we haven't changed much from our Stone Age ancestors who ate what they could in the late fall and winter because they never knew when their next hunt would take place, or whether it would be successful.

These old traits survive in us as unconscious habits. Maybe it's the cold and dark affecting our psyches. We tend to eat more in the winter and to gain weight—hopefully to lose it in the spring.

Now that we recognize the psychological component of winter weight gain, how can we outwit it? Dishes that need long cooking will soothe your inner caveperson without piling on the pounds. Try experimenting with soups, stews, and casseroles. The aromas of the long, slow cooking and the warmth of your kitchen will satisfy your emotional needs and help you avoid overeating.

283 THIS ADE WON'T HELP YOU ■ Orangeade, lemonade, and other fruit drinks sound "natural" and "healthy." But check their labeling. According to the U.S. Department of Agriculture, a fruit "ade" can contain as little as 15 percent fruit juice. The other 85 percent can be sugar and water, high-fructose corn syrup and water, or anything else. An 8-ounce serving often contains over 200 calories. Not the best choice for people with diabetes.

(And, of course, remember that as bad as fruit drinks are, drinking a lot of *pure* fruit juice isn't good for people with diabetes, either.)

Healthier choice: Eat a piece of fruit, drink lots of water, seltzer, or no-calorie flavored seltzer.

284 SUBSTITUTE OLIVES FOR CHIPS OR PRETZELS ■ Try olives when you're in the mood to snack on something that tastes salty. Although olives contain fat, it's monounsaturated, good for cardiovascular health. And the average green olive contains less than 10 calories, so it's better nutritionally than chips, which are often cooked in partially hydrogenated vegetable oil, or even pretzels, which contain mostly flour.

Besides, while many of us have devoured an entire bag of potato chips or pretzels at least once in our lives, who among us has wolfed down a whole bottle of olives?

285 PICKLES, TOO ■ Those little cornichons (baby pickles) that accompany pâté in good French restaurants can be nibbled on their own when you're in a snack mode. Most of them contain 5 calories or less, so they're truly a "free" food.

Other varieties of pickles are larger and contain more calories, but you're likely to be satisfied with fewer of them. Experiment with dill, sour, half-sour, mustard—all easy to find, all different, all tasty.

286 **PICK FROZEN PRODUCE . . . ■** Frozen fruits and vegetables are available all year 'round in your supermarket's freezer case. Because they are flash-frozen at the peak of ripeness, except for differences in texture, they are as tasty and nutritious as fresh produce. Possibly even more so, because they have been processed more quickly before being shipped.

287 **. . . AND FROZEN DESSERTS ■** While you're at the freezer case, check out the frozen desserts. You can enjoy many of them and still lose weight.

Among my favorites: No Sugar Added Fudgsicles (45 calories, 11 grams of carbohydrates), Tofutti Chocolate Fudge Treats (30 calories, 8 grams of carbohydrates), Yoplait Chocolate Mousse Fudge Bars (30 calories, 8 grams of carbohydrates), and Dole No Sugar Added, Tropicana Sugar-Free, and Welch's Sugar-Free fruit bars (25 calories, 6 grams of carbohydrates each).

288 **"IT'S ON SALE" IS NOT A GOOD ENOUGH REASON ■** Food manufacturers and supermarket chains spend billions of dollars a year to persuade you to buy their foods. No, it's not conspiracy theory—just the facts of life. One of their most profitable merchandising tools is the weekly flyer that highlights the foods that are on sale—complete with brightly colored pictures and juicy prices.

Fight back! Become a more educated consumer. Sale prices are not a good enough reason to buy specific foods, just as they're not a good enough reason to buy other merchandise you don't need.

Bonus: When you stop buying food just because it's on sale, you save money as well as losing weight.

289 **READ NEW FOOD CLAIMS CAREFULLY ■** Thanks to new, loosened U.S. Food and Drug Administration regulations, almost any food can claim almost any health benefit—regardless of any research—as long as the label uses such vague

"weasel words" as "evidence supports but is not conclusive," "bone strength," or "heart health." Skip the advertising claims, read the ingredients and their percentage of the adult RDA (Recommended Daily Allowance), then judge for yourself.

290 **REALLY KNOW HOW SWEET IT IS** ■ Food labeling is shown in grams, which doesn't help most Americans. We're still more comfortable with teaspoons.

Get a better idea of how sweet a packaged food is (and whether you should eat it) by using this formula: To calculate the number of teaspoons, divide the grams of carbohydrate or sugar by 4.2. Thus, a premium ice cream that contains 46 grams of carbohydrate in a half-cup serving has nearly 11 teaspoons of carbohydrate—mostly sugar—in that serving.

291 **PSYCH YOURSELF INTO VEGETABLES I: MAYBE YOU'RE A SUPERTASTER** ■ If you've hated vegetables since you were a kid, there's a good chance that you're a supertaster. This term is used to describe people who are extremely sensitive to bitter tastes because their tongues possess an unusually large number of taste buds.

It's not necessary to stick out your tongue and inspect it in the mirror. If you've always been a picky eater, turned down most vegetables, and asked for sauces and dressings on the side, you're most likely a supertaster.

As vegetables are so important in a healthful diet, read the tips in this section for ideas on how to make vegetables more palatable.

292 **PSYCH YOURSELF INTO VEGETABLES II: START WITH THE SWEET ONES** ■ Sweet vegetables have lots of vitamins and are easy to get used to. To make them even tastier, add grated orange rind, cinnamon, or ginger to carrots, sweet potatoes, or pumpkins, allspice to zucchini, and mint to green peas.

293 **PSYCH YOURSELF INTO VEGETABLES III: SEEK PERFECTION** ■ We've all experienced vegetables that weren't served at peak ripeness: woody asparagus, flabby tomatoes. No wonder they tasted terrible!

Other than growing your own and picking them just before dinner, your best bet is to buy produce in peak season at farmers' markets or greenmarkets. Spend some time chatting with the farmers and with fellow customers. Learn the characteristics of the most desirable vegetables and also how to store and prepare them. Admittedly, the best, freshest vegetables will be more expensive than the usual supermarket offerings, but you'll find them worth it.

294 **PSYCH YOURSELF INTO VEGETABLES IV: BAN BITTERNESS WITH BLANCHING** ■ Blanching vegetables before cooking them makes them much less bitter. This technique works especially well on cancer-fighting cruciferous vegetables: broccoli, brussels, cauliflower. Steam them for about a minute, then remove them and plunge them into cold water. This stops strong flavors from developing.

Tip: Use blanching to remove the skins from tomatoes.

295 **PSYCH YOURSELF INTO VEGETABLES V: BABIES MAY BE BETTER** ■ Baby vegetables usually have milder flavor; it gets stronger as they mature. And baby vegetables are more tender, so they require less cooking time. You can find them at farmers' markets or specialty grocers. Some baby vegetables are even available frozen.

296 **PSYCH YOURSELF INTO VEGETABLES VI: DRIZZLE WITH BUTTER OR OIL** ■ A teaspoon of butter or herb-infused olive oil won't wreck your diet and may persuade you to eat more vegetables because fat makes all food taste better. Even truffle-flavored olive oil can be an affordable treat one teaspoon at a time!

297 **PSYCH YOURSELF INTO VEGETABLES VII: SPRINKLE WITH CHEESE** ■ We're not talking your grandmother's heavy, fattening cheese sauce here! A teaspoon of crumbled blue cheese or grated Parmesan sprinkled over your vegetables can transform their taste.

298 **PSYCH YOURSELF INTO VEGETABLES VIII: SNEAK VEGGIES INTO OTHER DISHES** ■ Making an omelet? Throw in some cubed onions and green or red peppers. Top with sliced mushrooms. A meat loaf? Blend in a cup of grated onions or zucchini. Muffins? Some grated carrots or zucchini. Soups or stews? Let your imagination run wild. All of these contribute sneakily to the number of servings of vegetables to eat every day.

299 **PSYCH YOURSELF INTO VEGETABLES IX: ADD A LITTLE SPICE** ■ Have you always disliked spinach? Sprinkle it with nutmeg. Cabbage? Cook it with caraway seeds, mustard, or both. Kidney beans are the main ingredient in chili, so adding chili powder and cumin is a natural. Tomatoes are enhanced by many herbs and spices: basil, garlic, oregano, peppers of all types, and rosemary, for starters. Experiment!

300 **A LOW-FAT DIET MAY INCREASE THE RISK OF DIABETES** ■ A low-fat diet often leads to a greater consumption of carbohydrates—especially from refined flour—according to a recent Harvard School of Public Health Study of more than 42,000 men aged forty to seventy-five. The study suggested that such a high-carbohydrate diet could be worse for health than a higher-fat diet, as it increased the risk of diabetes.

Smarter choice: whole-grain products and healthful fats, like olive oil. (If this sounds like the "Mediterranean diet," you're right!)

301 CUSTOMIZE YOUR WEIGHT-LOSS PLAN ■ A session with a nutritionist may be just what you need to jump-start your weight-loss program. A good nutritionist will take a detailed medical and eating history and will ask pointed questions in order to design a weight-loss program that you will be more likely to stay on.

302 FOCUS ON WHAT YOU *CAN* EAT ■ The typical supermarket sells over 30,000 items, of which more than two-thirds are food. That's 20,000 choices. Even if you can't eat half of these, that still leaves you 10,000 foods you can choose from. You'll be more successful if you focus on what you *can* eat, not what you can't.

303 RECOGNIZE THAT OVERWEIGHT RUNS IN FAMILIES ■ Whether it's genetic or environmental—sharing the same menu, going back for second helpings—overweight runs in families.

Make weight loss run in your family instead. Get your family on a weight-loss program. Create your own in-house support system. You'll all benefit!

304 VISIT THE ETHNIC-FOODS SHELVES OF YOUR SUPERMARKET ■ The ethnic-foods shelves of your supermarket can surprise you with food choices you never thought of, in many combinations and sizes. Most supermarkets devote lots of space to Mexican and Asian cuisine. Browse here for interesting vegetable combinations, sauces, and seasonings.

305 TRACK YOUR SNACK ATTACKS ■ If you're having trouble losing weight, you may have selective amnesia about your visits to the refrigerator and pantry.

Here's an easy way to check: Start each day by putting a Post-It adhesive note and a pen on the refrigerator. Every time you open the fridge or go to the pantry, note the time and what you ate on the Post-It. When you go to bed, stick the Post-It in a notebook and date it. At the end of a week, you'll have an excellent record of when you're snacking, how much, and how you need to change your routine to break this habit.

306 SET UP LITTLE GOALS AND BIG ONES ∎ People who lose weight successfully choose both short-term and long-term goals. Losing fifty pounds is intimidating, but not if you start with a smaller, short-term goal of losing ten pounds in the first month, then five to ten pounds per month over the next four or five months. Setting and achieving goals one step at a time creates a feeling of accomplishment so that you're more likely to continue. Remember the old adage: "The journey of a thousand miles begins with a single step."

307 GOTTA BINGE? I: TRY THIS CATECHISM ∎ The urge to binge hits us all at one time or another. Here are some ways to deal with it:

Ask yourself: "On a scale of 1 to 5, with 5 being the maximum, how strong is this urge?" Be honest!
Ask yourself: "Can I wait ten minutes?" Set a kitchen timer for yourself.
Ask yourself: "If I knew that this binge would damage my eyes/kidneys/feet, would I still do it?" You probably wouldn't!

308 GOTTA BINGE? II: KEEP A "SAFE-SNACK" SHELF ∎ Having a "safe-snack" area that you have set aside in your refrigerator will minimize the effects of bingeing. Keep it generously stocked at all times so that you won't feel deprived.

What you put there depends on your food preferences. Here are some suggestions:

canned water-pack chicken breast or tuna
low-fat cheeses
hard-boiled eggs
cut-up vegetables
cherry tomatoes
mushrooms
tomato juice or vegetable juice
sugar-free Jell-O gelatin

309 **BINGE SUBSTITUTES I: SWEET** ■ So you crave something sweet.

You have lots of sugar-free, no-, and low-calorie choices. Among them: no-calorie soda and flavored seltzer, sugar-free Popsicles and fruit-juice pops, Fudgsicles, and Jell-O.

If it's chocolate you desire, try my recipes for guilt-free chocolate milk **(Tip No. 76)** or rum or cognac truffles **(Tip No. 78)**.

Or if you lust after apple pie, try my two quick apple-pie-substitute recipes **(Tips No. 162 and 163)**.

310 **BINGE SUBSTITUTES II: CREAMY** ■ So you crave something creamy. First, choose whether you want something sweet or something rich, like a high-fat cheese.

For something sweet, try my five Guilt-Free Cheesecake recipes at the end of this chapter.

For something rich, like Boursin, a garlic-herb cream-style cheese, make your own low-fat yogurt cheese **(Tip No. 165)**. Blend in garlic powder or slivered garlic, chives, parsley, and your favorite herbs after the whey has drained out of the yogurt.

311 **BINGE SUBSTITUTES III: SALTY** ■ Often it's the salt we really crave, rather than the pretzels or potato chips. If that's the case, skip the onion and sour-cream potato chips. Instead, try mixing onion salt into a cup of low-fat yogurt to achieve the same flavor.

For the crunch of pretzels with a little extra taste, grab a small handful of bacon-flavored soy bits. Or snack on a small dish of olives or pickles.

312 **FAST FOOD? CHECK ONLINE FIRST** ■ Fast food can still be an option if you do your homework first, rather than ordering impulsively without knowing the calorie, carbohydrate, fat, and protein content of your choice. Among the fast-food chains that post the nutritional content of their dishes online are Burger King, Hardee's, McDonald's, Ruby Tuesday, Subway, TGI Friday's, and Wendy's.

313 **SNACK ON SOY** ■ Soy snacks can be an excellent substitute for potato chips. Not only are they lower in calories and fat, but they also contain soy protein, which offers cardiovascular benefits by lowering cholesterol. Lots of flavor choices here, like barbecue, cheddar, nacho, ranch, and salt vinegar. For the best selection, try a large supermarket or health-food store.

314 **GOOD EATING HABITS MAKE YOU HEALTHIER THAN THE AVERAGE PERSON** ■ The silver lining in our diabetic cloud is that developing good eating habits and controlling our weight will make us healthier than the average person.

According to the U.S. Centers for Disease Control, about 60 percent of American adults are overweight, and many of them are obese. According to the World Health Organization, obesity is a worldwide epidemic. And obesity is linked to many other diseases: cardiovascular, hypertension, stroke, and joint problems for starters.

Eating sensibly and carefully can put us ahead of the average American, who doesn't. For firsthand empirical evidence, just look at the contents of the shopping carts on your next trip to the supermarket.

315 **YOU MAY DO BETTER ON SIX LITTLE MEALS A DAY** ■ If you are not losing weight on three meals a day, you may do better on five or six smaller meals. Some nutritionists believe that people burn more calories when they eat more frequently and their metabolic furnace is always burning food.

Remember: You can't eat more calories, you just have to divide them differently—with a smaller breakfast, lunch, and dinner, and midmorning, afternoon, and bedtime snacks.

316

COCOA LOWERS CANCER RISK ■ Diabetes increases cancer risk. Now there's a tasty way to lower it:

Here's a good reason to enjoy your morning or evening cocoa. Cornell University researchers discovered that a cup of hot cocoa (pure cocoa powder and water) contains twice the quantity of phenolic phytochemicals—powerful cancer-fighting antioxidants—found in a glass of red wine, three times the quantity found in a cup of green tea, and five times the quantity found in a cup of black tea. The antioxidants protect against cancer by ridding the body of damaging free radicals.

Note: Previous research suggests that adding milk to the cocoa could block its antioxidant action.

317

VARIETY IS THE KEY TO YOUR WEIGHT-LOSS SUCCESS ■ Let's face it: Most diets fail because they are too restrictive and boring. Eventually dieters cry: "Let me outta here!" But if you can choose from among hundreds of healthful foods prepared in many different ways, you actually have *thousands* of possibilities, even if you're a picky eater.

When you realize the vast number of your options, you are much more likely to stick with your diet—or even rotate among weight-loss programs after a few months or so—and keep on losing weight!

318

STEAM—DON'T MICROWAVE—YOUR VEGGIES ■ Produce loses as much as 97 percent of its flavonoids, a type of potent antioxidant, when it is microwaved, according to a recent research study from the Department of Food Technology, a major research center in Murcia, Spain. Microwaving destroyed the highest percentage of flavonoids, followed by conventional boiling.

Steaming preserved almost all the flavonoids, so steam your veggies or eat them raw for maximum nutrition.

319 FIVE-POUND WEIGHT SWINGS ARE MEANINGLESS ■

Don't panic if your weight fluctuates from day to day. Weight swings of five pounds have no significance because they can be caused by water retention and many other factors. In fact, the five-pound weight swings can occur if you weigh yourself three or four times a day, as many dieters do.

You can get a better sense of whether you're losing weight by weighing yourself only once a week—or even once a month.

320 DON'T HIDE FROM YOUR SCALE ■ Not weighing

yourself at all is just as self-destructive as weighing yourself after every time you go to the bathroom. Not weighing yourself for weeks or months makes you the king or queen of denial. Psychologists call this hiding from the scale "avoidance behavior": You don't want to be confronted by the cold, hard numbers showing how much you've overeaten.

Instead, use your scale as a helpful tool to keep you focused on your weight-loss program and all the advantages your weight loss will give you.

321 DINE TO SLOW MUSIC ■ Listening to sweet, stately

music when you eat slows you down. You relax, take more time at the table, but actually eat less while enjoying it more.

Here's the science behind it: We speed up unconsciously to fast music, and dawdle to slow music. Eating more slowly gives our brains the time to signal our stomachs that we are full.

Try chamber music, opera or ballet music, symphonic works by the great classical masters from your own library or classical FM stations.

322

FORM A LUNCH BUNCH ■ If you have congenial coworkers who enjoy tasting new foods, try this:

For a group of five, choose one person to bring lunch for everyone on Monday, another person on Tuesday, and so on. Discuss food preferences so that everyone will be able to eat something every day, and nobody will feel unhappy.

This lunch club will save all of you lots of money and time. If you go for a walk after lunch, you'll burn some extra calories, too.

■

IN THE SPIRIT and intent of *1,001 Tips for Living Well with Diabetes,* I end this chapter with several recipes for "guilt-free" cheesecakes.

Rich, creamy, not too sweet. Cheesecake is a favorite dessert that dieters hate to deny themselves. But a portion of plain Cheesecake Factory cheesecake contains a whopping 710 calories, 49 grams of carbohydrate, and 49 grams of fat. Fruit-flavored cheesecakes are even more fattening.

OK, I admit that the recipes that follow have no crusts. But that's where the calories and carbohydrates lurk and—let's face it—the appeal of cheesecake is *not* in the crust.

What you'll find here are recipes ranging from as little as 91 calories to a maximum of 190 calories per serving, with 5–17 grams of carbohydrate, 2–7 grams of fat, and as much as 22 grams of protein per serving.

Enjoy them!

323

GUILT-FREE CHEESECAKE I: COEUR À LA CRÈME (SERVES 2) ■

1 cup low-fat cottage cheese
2 oz. Neufchâtel cheese, slightly softened
pinch of salt
several envelopes Equal or Splenda, to taste
1 cup fresh strawberries, raspberries, or blueberries

▶ Thorougly blend all ingredients except berries in a bowl. Refrigerate.

▶ About 15 minutes before serving, form the cheese into a heart shape, place on a pretty serving platter, and surround with berries.

Approximately 190 calories, 12 grams carbohydrate (mostly from the berries), 7 grams of fat, and 19 grams of protein per serving.

324 GUILT-FREE CHEESECAKE II: MASCARPONE WITH APRICOTS OR PEACHES (SERVES 4 TO 6) ■ Mascarpone, named after the eponymous Italian cream cheese, is a more sybaritic version of Coeur à la Crème.

4 oz. whipped low-fat cottage cheese
4 oz. Neufchâtel cheese, slightly softened
¼ cup plain low-fat yogurt
several envelopes Equal or Splenda, to taste
2 tbsp. Grand Marnier, cognac, or light rum
fresh apricot or peach halves

▶ Combine all ingredients except fruit in a large bowl. Beat until well blended. Mound in a cone on a pretty serving dish and surround with the apricot or peach halves.
▶ Spoon a little of the cheese mixture into the fruit half and eat.

Based on 4 servings, approximately 136 calories, 6 grams of carbohydrate, 7 grams of fat, and 9 grams of protein per serving. Three apricots per serving add 51 calories and 12 grams of carbohydrate; one peach adds 37 calories and 10 grams of carbohydrate.

325 GUILT-FREE CHEESECAKE III: LEMON CHEESECAKE (SERVES 4) ■

2 large eggs
2 cup low-fat cottage cheese
2 tsp. vanilla extract
1 tsp. lemon extract

2 tbsp. fresh lemon juice
2 tbsp. nonfat milk powder
1 envelope Equal or Splenda
2 egg whites
pinch cream of tartar (optional)
butter-flavored vegetable spray

▶ Preheat oven to 350 degrees.
▶ Mix all ingredients except egg whites and cream of tartar in a large bowl. Beat egg whites and cream of tartar until stiff peaks form, then fold into other ingredients.
▶ Pour into springform pan greased with butter-flavored vegetable spray. Bake for 30–35 minutes. Cool. Refrigerate overnight. Before serving, garnish with grated lemon peel, if desired.

Approximately 151 calories, 5 grams carbohydrate, 4 grams fat, 22 grams protein per serving.

326 GUILT-FREE CHEESECAKE IV: STRAWBERRY CHEESECAKE (SERVES 2) ■

2 tsp. sugar-free strawberry Jell-O
1 tbsp. hot water
1 cup strawberries, reserving several of the prettiest for garnish
⅔ cup low-fat cottage cheese
1 large egg white
1 tsp. almond extract

▶ Dissolve Jell-O in hot water. Blend strawberries and cottage cheese in blender, then add Jell-O mixture.
▶ Beat egg white until stiff. Add almond extract to berry mixture. Fold in egg white. Chill in a serving bowl until set and garnish with remaining strawberries.

Variation: Substitute sugar-free raspberry Jell-O, raspberries, and vanilla extract.

Approximately 91 calories, 7 grams carbohydrate, less than 1 gram fat, and 4 grams protein for either version.

327 GUILT-FREE CHEESECAKE V: CHERRY CHEESECAKE (SERVES 8) ■

3 large eggs, separated
1 lb. farmer cheese or pot cheese
4 envelopes Equal or Splenda
½ tsp. vanilla extract
¼ tsp. cinnamon

Cherry Glaze
1 large can water-packed black cherries, pitted
1 tbsp. cornstarch
1 envelope Equal or Splenda
few drops red food coloring

▶ If you can't find either farmer or pot cheese, you'll need to start this recipe a day early. Put 1½ lbs. of low-fat cottage cheese in a very fine sieve placed over a bowl, and put it in the refrigerator. The whey (liquid) will drain into the bowl, leaving you with the pot cheese.
▶ Preheat oven to 325 degrees.
▶ Place egg yolks and other ingredients in blender. Blend at low speed until smooth.
▶ Meanwhile, beat egg whites until peaks form.
▶ Place cheese mixture into a bowl and gently fold in egg whites.
▶ Pour mixture into a springform pan greased with butter-flavored vegetable spray. Bake 15 minutes.
▶ Turn oven up to 450 degrees and bake 5 minutes more. Remove cake from oven and prepare Cherry Glaze.
▶ Drain cherries, reserving liquid. Add cornstarch and mix until well blended. Heat mixture over medium flame until it starts simmering and is slightly thickened. Remove from

flame, add sugar substitute and food coloring, and mix thoroughly.

▶ Place the cherries on top of the cheesecake and spoon the glaze over them. Refrigerate the cake in the springform pan for several hours to overnight before unmolding and serving.

▶ The glaze firms as it chills.

Approximately 92 calories, 9 grams carbohydrate, 2 grams fat, and 9 grams protein per serving.

3

Working with Your Doctors and Other Health-Care Professionals

328 BE A "GOOD" PATIENT ■ "Good" by *our* standards, not theirs. This is *not* the same as taking your doctor's every word as gospel.

Bring a list of questions to every appointment. Keep a log of your blood-glucose readings and bring that, too. Show that you are very motivated about preventing serious complications; some diabetics aren't.

Let your doctor know that you won't pester him/her, but if you phone, it means that you're in *serious* trouble and need a quick callback or appointment. Suggest this as a "treatment contract."

Ideally —especially if you are insulin-dependent—your doctor will let you fax weekly logs and then call you if there are unusual readings or patterns, or your medication needs adjusting. As a result, you probably will have fewer extreme high and low blood-glucose readings.

329 MAKE SURE YOUR DOCTOR TAKES YOUR MEDICAL HISTORY AND ORDERS A C-PEPTIDE TEST ■ Every competent doctor will ask you to provide a complete family medical history. But in the case of diabetes, both type 1 and type 2 can manifest in the same families. Many doctors will not necessarily order a C-peptide test, which measures how much insulin your body produces, and thus will determine whether you have type 1 or type 2 diabetes. Even though the treatments for type 1 and type 2 can be similar, and thus doctors may feel this information is not essential, request it as part of your treatment so that you know for sure, from the beginning, which condition you have.

330
DON'T ACCEPT BAD MEDICAL CARE ■ An endocrinologist I saw—once—broke off our examination to see a drug-company salesman. As I waited for him to return, my blood glucose tanked and I started getting hypoglycemic symptoms.

When he came back and I told him what was happening, he started chewing me out.

Not only did I never see him again, but I told my family doctor and also wrote to the medical group's president. That endocrinologist is not working at the medical group anymore, and now I have an excellent endocrinologist at that group.

331
TESTING, TESTING ■ You should have these lab tests done at least once a year. If your doctor doesn't order them, ask why.

▶ CBC (Complete Blood Count)—This test measures the number of red and white blood cells, whether there are any abnormalities in the types of white blood cells (eosinophils, basophils, neutrophils, lymphocytes, immature "stab" cells), and hemoglobin levels, which diagnose anemia.

▶ Urine microalbumin—This test checks the presence of the protein albumin and determines how well your kidneys are functioning.

▶ Creatinine, BUN (Blood Urea Nitrogen)—This is another test of how well your kidneys are functioning and preventing the buildup of toxins.

▶ Lipid profile—This test checks the levels of fats in your blood, which can be a precursor of heart attacks and strokes.

▶ Liver profile—Because the liver is the major cleansing organ of the body, this test measures liver function, which can be affected by toxins—especially from drugs you are taking.

These tests should be done every three months:

▶ Fasting blood glucose—This test checks whether your fasting blood-glucose levels are too high, too low, or within normal range, and tells your doctor whether your medication needs to be adjusted.
▶ Glycohemoglobin A1C—Like Santa Claus coming to town, this test tells your doctor how "good" (good control) or "bad" (poor control) your blood glucose has been for the past three months, with an emphasis on the last month. There's no way to "cheat" on this test.

332 **SHARE INFORMATION WITH YOUR DOCTORS** ■ *You* have more time to read about new research and treatment for diabetes than your family doctor, who has to spread reading time over many medical topics, or even your endocrinologist, who has to read about thyroid, parathyroid, and adrenal problems, too.

Web sites for the *New England Journal of Medicine* and *The Lancet* are especially good sources. So are search engines and even the Tuesday "Science Times" section of the *New York Times* and the "Trends and Innovations" column of *Investor's Business Daily.*

Your doctors will appreciate your help and will likely give you better care.

333 **OTHER SPECIALISTS YOU SHOULD SEE** ■ Get referrals from your family doctor or endocrinologist if you need to, but see these specialists:

Cardiologist—every six months or more often if you're on medication.

Ophthalmologist—every six months to catch glaucoma, retinopathy, and other diabetic eye diseases at their earliest stages.
Podiatrist—as needed.

334

CITE A "HIGHER AUTHORITY" ■ Unfortunately, many family doctors and nurses are very ignorant about diabetes.

Here are some horror stories from fellow diabetics:

"I had a general-practice doctor tell me I was obsessive/compulsive before I was rushed to the hospital with a blood-glucose reading over 900!"

"A doctor told me to take insulin when my blood glucose was low. I had sugar pills ripped out of my hands while on the verge of passing out (from hypoglycemia)."

"I said a (hypoglycemic) reaction was coming on. I was asked to make it wait."

To tactfully educate these "medical experts" while protecting your health and sanity, cite a "higher authority." For example: "Doctor, did you know that the American Diabetes Association/Joslin Diabetes Center says that diabetics should have juice/sugar and water/regular soda when their blood glucose is low—not insulin?"

I hope that the ADA and Joslin won't mind!

335

ASK YOUR DOCTOR TO CHECK YOUR BLOOD PRESSURE AT EVERY VISIT ■ If your blood pressure is high at the beginning of the examination, ask to have it checked at the end, too. Many people who test high at the beginning because they're nervous or worried relax toward the end of the examination, so the reading is more accurate.

Diabetics are susceptible to many kinds of circulatory problems, so your doctor should keep a record of all your blood-pressure readings.

336

CHECK YOUR BLOOD PRESSURE FREQUENTLY, TOO ■ You really don't need your own blood-pressure monitor unless you suffer from high blood pressure. (Many diabetics do.) Most pharmacies have a blood-pressure testing station, and you can check your blood pressure easily just by putting your arm into a sleeve that inflates automatically and then displays your blood pressure and heart rate.

Many pharmacies provide small cards on which you can keep a log of eight or ten blood-pressure readings that you can bring or send to your doctor.

337 **GET YOUR FLU SHOT AS EARLY AS POSSIBLE** ■ You can't afford to overlook this crucial annual ritual. People with diabetes are six times as likely to be hospitalized if they develop influenza as people without diabetes. This is a risk you can't afford to take.

338 **BEFORE GASTRIC-BYPASS SURGERY, ASK YOUR DOCTOR ABOUT ALTERNATIVES** ■ Many doctors will prescribe gastric-bypass surgery for their patients who are extremely overweight or obese. Overweight is defined as 10 to 20 percent higher than the normal weight, as defined in standard height-weight tables. Obese is defined as 20 percent higher than normal weight for men, 25 percent higher for women. Morbid (life-threatening) obesity is defined as more than 100 pounds overweight. A good Web site for weight tables is www.healthchecksystems.com/heightweightchart.htm.

If your doctor recommends gastric-bypass surgery and your medical insurance will pay for it, ask your doctor about the alternatives, which are both less risky and far less expensive. Gastric-bypass surgery can cost from $20,000 to $40,000. In contrast, the weight-loss programs at Duke University and the Joslin Diabetes Center cost only about 10 percent of that amount.

In late 2003, the program at Duke cost about $4,295 for one week and $5,395 for two weeks, but seasonal discounts bring those rates down to $3,500 and $3,895, plus $60–$70 per night for your room.

Joslin's Do-It (Diabetes Outpatient Intensive Treatment) lasts only three and one-half days, but is truly intensive, starting at approximately 7:00 AM and running past dinner. Costs run $2,472 to $3,602, plus your room at a nearby motel.

Insurance companies should be delighted to pay all your expenses because they are so much lower than the costs of the gastric-bypass surgery. Even more important, in most cases you will be better off learning successful new behaviors to help you lose weight and improve your health than undergoing the surgery and enduring the long-term side effects.

339 ON MEDICARE? YOU CAN STILL FIND A GOOD DOCTOR ■ Many doctors limit the number of Medicare patients they accept because reimbursement payments are so low, but these strategies may work for you:

Mention the name of the person who referred you. The doctor may accept you as a patient to avoid alienating the colleague or patient who referred you.

State that you are looking for a permanent doctor. Doctors prefer regular patients to acute-care patients.

Tell the doctor if your Medicare plan is fee-for-service rather than managed care. Reimbursement payments are higher, so the doctor will be more likely to take you on as a patient.

Even if you are turned down once, try again—especially early in the year. After reviewing their books at the end of the year, many doctors decide to accept new patients.

340 MAKE YOUR DOCTOR'S STAFF PART OF YOUR TEAM ■ Your doctor's employees are gatekeepers. They control access to your doctor. They can facilitate or roadblock your appointments and do you lots of small favors if they like you.

Case in point: A friend was able to get a flu shot immediately, rather than having to make an appointment for a separate visit several weeks later. My friend got special treatment because several months ago she asked the nurse, "Are you having a bad day? You look tired."

Treat your doctor's staff with TLC. Remember their names and little bits of personal information. Are they married? Do they have children?

Are they planning a vacation? Bring them a small Christmas or Hanukkah present. You'll be glad you did when you need that emergency or add-on appointment!

341 GET WHAT YOU NEED FROM YOUR INSURANCE COMPANY ■ Are you having problems getting enough supplies to test your blood glucose as frequently as necessary to keep your glycohemoglobin A1C low? Is your doctor having problems getting authorization for your supplies? Here's how to get what you need:

Most private insurance plans have a case manager who can approve individual patient requests based on special needs. Contact the case manager and explain your treatment regimen and the supplies you need that will keep you out of hospitals and emergency rooms. Ask the case manager what documentation is needed and get the case manager that documentation.

Keep on pushing for what you need. Some states are trying to pass legislation allowing insurance plans to refuse coverage for diabetes supplies. *Don't let this happen!*

342 STICK WITH ONE PHARMACY ■ When you use only one pharmacy, your pharmacist has a record of *all* the drugs you are taking and can alert you about any potential drug interactions or side effects. (It's also a lot more convenient.)

343 USE A PHARMACY WITH A GOOD COMPUTER SYSTEM ■ Most chain pharmacies (and many smaller ones) print out and attach very complete drug information with every prescription.

A typical printout will include instructions on using the drug, side effects, precautions (e.g., previous allergic reactions and diseases, use during pregnancy or nursing), interactions with other drugs, what to do if you have missed a dose or have overdosed accidentally, and how to store the drug.

Keep these printouts handy for future reference. Do not discard them.

344 **HAVE YOUR PHARMACIST SUBSTITUTE SMALLER NEEDLES** ■ Always ask your pharmacist to give you the smallest-gauge-needle insulin syringe available. In general, your pharmacist will not substitute a *shorter* needle than what your doctor has prescribed, but will substitute a thinner one. The smaller gauge doesn't cost more money, and you will certainly notice the difference in comfort.

345 **GET COPIES OF YOUR MEDICAL RECORDS** ■ Ask every doctor's assistant or receptionist for a copy of your medical record—and make sure that you get it. Build a file that you can refer to again and again and research whatever diagnosis and treatment that you may not understand. Use it to develop questions for your next visit to this doctor, or to other specialists. Use it to monitor your progress.

346 **TIME YOUR LAB TESTS** ■ Get your lab tests done two weeks before your doctor's appointment so that they'll be ready for your doctor to review before the appointment.

347 **THAT ALL-IMPORTANT BLOOD-GLUCOSE DIARY** ■ Bring at least two weeks of your blood-glucose diary to your doctor's appointment. (Three weeks' worth is more useful if you have the time.) Write down the time of each test and the result, the timing, name, and dosage of any diabetes drugs you are taking, and any unusually heavy meals or exercise. The more complete your diary is, the more your doctor will be able to advise you.

I keep the original of this diary, make a photocopy for my doctor, and bring both to every appointment. That way I can write his comments on my copy and refer to it at home.

348   **YOUR Q&A NOTEBOOK** ■ A 4" x 6" notebook can be an invaluable tool in your medical care.

For each doctor you see, keep a running list of questions and symptoms, with dates. The best way to do this is to use a double-page spread with your questions on the right-hand page. Save the left-hand page for your doctor's answers to your questions.

For example, you might list:

Blood pressure?
Results of lab tests?
Adjust drugs? New prescriptions
11/2 Pain in right toes—arthritis or neuropathy? Treatment?

Keep a different double-page for each doctor, marking the top with his/her name, specialty, and appointment date. Make a duplicate copy when you have time, and tell a family member or friend where it is and to bring it if you should need a hospital or emergency room.

349   **TRY A "GROUP APPOINTMENT"** ■ One of the newest trends in patient care is the "group appointment," in which several patients share long group appointments—as opposed to short, hard-to-schedule private appointments—and have a chance to ask all the questions that they want to.

This may work especially well for people with diabetes. Talk with your doctor about the possibilities.

350   **YOUR FRIENDLY *NEIGHBORHOOD* DOCTOR** ■ Several times in the last ten or twelve years (I've had diabetes for sixteen), I have owed my health—and avoided a trip to the emergency room—to a doctor who was a neighbor.

Of course it's Murphy's Law that we come down with a strep throat on Friday night or Saturday morning, after regular doctors' office hours. So having a friend who lives nearby who will write that all-important prescription on a weekend—so that you can fill it immediately—can be a godsend.

351

THE BEST TIME FOR APPOINTMENTS ■ Do you hate to wait? These are the best times for doctors' appointments, when you're least likely to cool your heels in the waiting room.

If you hate to wait, be the first appointment in the morning, or the first one after lunch. Call before you leave to check if the doctor is running late.

To guarantee *your* choice of appointments, make follow-up appointments before you leave the doctor's office. Even if your next visit isn't for many months, you'll have your choice of a pretty empty schedule, and you won't waste time later calling for an appointment.

352

HAVING DIABETES DOES NOT EXEMPT YOU FROM OTHER DISEASES ■ Sad but true, having diabetes may actually increase the likelihood that you have other problems: cardiovascular, vision, and others. Simply getting older brings still other diseases, like arthritis.

This means multiple doctors' appointments, but look on the bright side: Being aggressive about your medical care can prevent or delay hospitalization, and can extend your life.

353

DOUBLE UP YOUR APPOINTMENTS ■ Because more than one doctor is taking care of you, if you belong to a medical group, it's smart to double up on your appointments. For example, see one doctor at 9:00 and another at 10:30 or 11:00 on the same day. You'll save both traveling time and time off from work.

354 **TWO REASONS TO DUMP YOUR DOCTOR** ■ Fast and furious:

(1) being put on hold for fifteen minutes.
(2) not having your phone call returned in twenty-four hours.
No excuses—you are the customer, and *you are important.*

355 **IS YOUR DOCTOR BOARD CERTIFIED?** ■ Doctors who have been practicing for more than three years should be certified by a medical board in their specialty. This certification goes beyond an M.D. It is more like a postgraduate degree and is granted by one of the twenty-four medical boards that are members of the American Board of Medical Specialties. Most boards have certification, recertification, and maintenance certification programs to keep their doctors current in the latest developments in medicine.

You can check whether your doctors have been board certified by calling toll-free (866) 275-2267, or logging on to www.abms.org, which has links to its twenty-four member boards.

Note: Endocrinologists are certified by the American Board of Internal Medicine.

356 **YOU MAY BE COVERED FOR ALTERNATIVE-MEDICINE SERVICES** ■ Many insurance companies are now covering such alternative-medicine services as acupuncture, massage therapy/bodywork, nutritional counseling, and mind-body relaxation treatments. Depending on your policy, these services may be discounted, or you may have to make a copayment. It's worth checking!

357 **GET THE MOST ACCURATE BLOOD-PRESSURE READING** ■ Blood pressure is important because people with diabetes are so susceptible to cardiovascular problems.

Ask your doctor to measure the pressure in both arms, not just one.

Lower pressure in one arm could mean that your arteries may be partially blocked on that side and need to be checked further.

358 **FIND A DOCTOR WHO'S FLEXIBLE** ■ You'll do better with a doctor who doesn't impose a rigid one-size-fits-all mind-set on your treatment. You want, need, and deserve a doctor who will be responsive and who will tailor a treatment program to your individual situation. Someone who will keep tweaking and fine-tuning your medications until they are the best possible fit.

359 **HAVE YOUR DOCTOR CHECK YOUR BLOOD-GLUCOSE METER** ■ At least once a year, bring your blood-glucose meter, test strips, and lancet to your doctor's appointment and ask him to test your blood glucose on your meter and on the meter in his office. Very often there are significant differences in the numbers, and you will manage your diabetes better if you work with a meter that is accurate.

It's much better to test your meter against the lab's results. The doctor's meter might not be any more accurate than yours, and many doctors and nurses aren't very sophisticated about meter technology.

360 **AFFORDABLE HEALTH INSURANCE I: FORM YOUR OWN TINY CORPORATION OR BUSINESS ALLIANCE** ■ In many states, even a group of two people qualifies and can get a policy with premiums that are 20 to 50 percent less than individual policies. Usually, each person must work at least twenty-five hours a week and pay Social Security taxes.

361 **AFFORDABLE HEALTH INSURANCE II: JOIN AN ASSOCIATION THAT OFFERS GROUP COVERAGE** ■ Many professional and trade associations, alumni, religious, and service organizations offer group coverage. (In fact, I joined an authors' organization in order to obtain affordable medical insurance.) Try a trade association, Chamber of Commerce, Rotary, Kiwanis, or these: AARP (800) 523-5800, www.aarp.org, National Association for the Self-Employed (800) 232-6273, www.nase.org, or United Service Association for Health Care (800) 872-1187, www.usahc.com. If you are in the U.S. military or are a family member, try USAA (800) 365-8722, www.usaa.com.

362 AFFORDABLE HEALTH INSURANCE III: IF YOU MUST GET AN INDIVIDUAL POLICY ■ Use a health-insurance broker to help find the best policy for your needs. Here are some sources: National Association of Health Underwriters (703) 276-0220, www.nahu.ora. Digital Insurance (888) 470-2121, www.digital-insurance.com, and eHealth Insurances Services (800) 977-8860, www.ehealthinsurance.com.

363 BETTER DOCTOR-PATIENT COMMUNICATION I: BE AN INDIVIDUAL ■ With many doctors treating as many as one hundred patients a week, your first job is to remind your doctor who you are, especially if you're a fairly new patient.

Make eye contact with your doctor and make sure there's a response. Then tell your doctor about what's been happening in your life since the last visit. (Your doctor should be taking notes.)

364 BETTER DOCTOR-PATIENT COMMUNICATION II: OPENING THE WINDOW ■ When you discuss your blood-glucose log and food diary with your doctor, focus your questions: "Do you see any patterns here? Has anything changed? Should I do anything differently?"

These questions open a dialogue in which new information can be exchanged. For example, your insulin dosage may need to be tweaked very slightly; adding or subtracting only one unit can make a big difference in your blood-glucose control.

It goes without saying that doctors work harder for motivated patients. You want to be one of them!

365 **DOCTOR-PATIENT COMMUNICATION III: DISCUSS FUTURE GOALS ■** At every visit, ask your doctor, "What do I need to improve? Is there anything new or different I should try?" This is especially important if you have type 2 diabetes because, according to an article in the January 2002 issue of the *Southern Medical Journal*, a study found that "internal medicine physicians have negative attitudes toward type 2 diabetes that require future educational interventions."

366 **BETTER DOCTOR-PATIENT COMMUNICATION IV: GET IN THE LOOP ■** Ask your doctor to e-mail you between your visits if there are important new developments in diabetes care. Medical conferences take place year-round, and many medical journals are published weekly or monthly. You want to stay current so that you can take the best care of your diabetes.

367 **ENLARGE YOUR HEALTH-CARE TEAM ■** Besides your primary-care doctor and your ophthalmologist, get referrals to these other professionals if you have more specific problems: an endocrinologist specializing in diabetes care and a dietitian or Certified Diabetes Educator. Many medical groups and communities also offer diabetes classes and support groups.

368 **ADD A PHYSIATRIST TO YOUR TEAM ■** Physiatry (the practice of physical and rehabilitation medicine) is a fairly new specialty. It covers the musculoskeletal system, so it can be useful in treating many joint and muscle problems without your having to resort to surgery. My personal opinion: I would see a physiatrist first, then a surgeon if rehabilitation treatments didn't work well enough.

369

DOCTOR BILLS: LET'S MAKE A DEAL ■ You can often negotiate lower fees with doctors, dentists, hospitals, and pharmacies.

Do a little homework first: Learn how much health insurance companies and Medicare are paying for the same services. In general, managed-care companies receive a 40 percent discount on medical services, and doctors will often give you a similar discount.

Start by asking the doctor, "Can you help me out? Could you please bill me what Medicare or insurance companies pay you?"

4

Avoiding/Surviving Hospital and Emergency Rooms

370 **KNOW YOUR BLOOD TYPE** ■ When you are in the hospital or emergency room, crucial time can be wasted if your blood must be typed before you receive a transfusion. If you don't know your blood type, ask your doctor to run the proper tests at your next visit.

Make sure that you know your family members' blood types and that they know yours.

371 **WEAR A MEDICAL IDENTIFICATION BRACELET AT ALL TIMES** ■ For clear identification that this is more than just jewelry, your bracelet should have the caduceus—the international medical symbol—on it, and the words "diabetic" or "insulin," and your blood type. (You can buy these at pharmacies or have them made to order.)

372 **. . . AND CARRY A MEDICAL ID CARD IN YOUR WALLET** ■ The card will have much more information. Many cards enclose a microfilm chip that displays your personal medical profile and treatment authorization. It tells medical personnel to use an ophthalmoscope or a microfilm reader to view your medical history, allergies, blood type, treatment authorization, medical coverage, person to notify, and many other vital facts to help medical personnel diagnose your needs in a medical emergency.

Emergency Medical Service and emergency-room workers are trained to search for this card if you are unconscious.

373 **KEEP A MEDICATION LIST** ■ Have a list of all medications that you are taking, and their dosages. If your doctor changes a medication or dosage, update your list immediately. Keep a copy of this list with you at all times so that you will have it in an emergency. *If you don't have any place to keep this list on your trip to the emergency room, then pin it to whatever you are wearing.*

You will also help your doctors—and yourself—if you include the name of your family physician and his phone number, as well as the name and phone number of the doctor who prescribed each medication.

374 **LIST YOUR ALLERGIES** ■ Make a list of all your allergies (food, pollen, pets, et al.), as well as any prescription and nonprescription drugs to which you are allergic. Keep it with you or put it with other medical papers that you take to the hospital.

375 **BRING YOUR INSURANCE CARDS** ■ Be sure to take with you any membership cards of major medical plans, HMOs and/or Medicare, Medicaid, and AARP.

376 **WRITE DOWN ALL YOUR SYMPTOMS** ■ As best you can, regardless of the physical and mental pain and stress you are suffering, try to write down every single symptom you are experiencing and how it may relate to an already existing condition that has caused you problems before this. Unless you write down all of this, you may forget to tell the doctor the one clue that would lead to an accurate diagnosis.

377

BRING A RELATIVE OR FRIEND WITH YOU ■ You may be in too much pain, or may not be coherent or conscious. Having someone with you to deal with medical personnel and hospital procedures can make you feel much less frightened and much more comfortable.

378

KNOW HOW EMERGENCY ROOMS WORK ■ Most emergency rooms operate on a two-track system. Patients who are seriously in need of immediate and possibly lifesaving treatment get to see a doctor first. This system is called triage, familiar to us *M*A*S*H* fans. Many hospitals also use the "fast-track system," which gets patients who need minimal attention for minor ailments and injuries in and out of the emergency room as quickly as possible.

Unless you are put on triage or on the fast-track system, the chances are that you will probably have to wait for medical attention an hour or two, or even longer. To make the waiting easier and less nerve-racking, take along some light reading, a few magazines, or a book of crossword puzzles to help you pass the time.

379

DOCTOR'S ORDERS CAN RAISE YOUR COMFORT LEVEL ■ Have your admitting doctor write orders stating that you have permission to test your own blood glucose, take your own medications, and order your own meals—especially if your hospitalization is not connected to your diabetes.

380

PLAN FOR AUTOLOGOUS TRANSFUSION ■ Is elective surgery in your future? Then plan for autologous (your own blood) transfusion in case you need blood.

This is how it works: First ask your surgeon whether your surgery might *even remotely* necessitate a transfusion, and how many pints of blood you might need. Then ask your surgeon what the guidelines are for your donating blood for your own use.

In general, you will have to go to your hospital's blood bank every two weeks to donate a pint of blood at each appointment. You will need to drink extra liquid, load up on iron-rich foods, and even take an iron supplement to make sure that you are not anemic and will not develop anemia before surgery.

Transfusion using your own blood guarantees that there will be no errors in cross-matching and that the donor is free of disease.

What happens if you don't need a transfusion? Then the hospital uses your blood for other purposes. What's crucial: *You have eliminated a major potential risk.*

381
MUNCHIES ON YOUR BEDSIDE TABLE LURE DOCTORS AND NURSES ■ If you want to guarantee that doctors and nurses visit you frequently, keep cookies or candy on your bedside table. It's a lot more convenient for them than the hospital cafeteria or the nearest vending machine, and their frequent visits will give you or members of your family the opportunity to ask questions and get answers, or just get more water, pain pills, or get your pillows fluffed.

382
WEAR GOGGLES WHEN WORKING WITH TOOLS ■ If you are working in your house or garden, wear protective goggles. Rust specks that get into your eyes can send you to the emergency room in extreme pain and with possible cornea damage. Regular eyeglasses aren't safe enough because they don't offer protection on the sides.

383
AVOID SPLINTERS—ESPECIALLY DANGEROUS FOR DIABETICS ■ Splinters can get infected easily. Splinters in your feet are especially dangerous because feet contain lots of sweat glands that create an ideal warm, moist environment for germs to multiply.

To avoid nasty splinters, wear shoes when you are in your yard or on a wooden deck. Wear gloves when you are working with wood or metal, or are in your garden.

384 **STAY AWAY FROM HOSPITALS AND EMERGENCY ROOMS IN JULY** ■ These newbies may have graduated medical school and earned the right to put "M.D." after their names, but internship is their first real experience with patients.

If you can, wait until October, when the new interns have had several months of seasoning—on other patients.

385 **PACK NOW FOR LATER** ■ Anyone who thinks he might ever need an emergency room should pack a small bag now. A small canvas bag with your insurance information, a book or magazine, a list of all medications and vitamins or herbs you take, an acceptable snack and a bottle of water, important friends' or relatives' numbers to call, and a change of underwear are wise inclusions. Just like an expectant mother's "It's time, honey" bag, yours should be immediately grabbable and should contain all the necessary and desirable things you'll wish you had with you—either as you are hurried into an ambulance, or as you sit and pick your cuticles in the waiting room outside the ER.

386 **SAVE THE ANTIBACTERIAL SOAP FOR SPECIAL OCCASIONS** ■ All the antibacterial detergents and soaps being sold today have their effect on bacteria: the few that survive are breeding more resistant strains. It's not necessary—in fact, it's not preferable—to use anything stronger than regular soaps or detergents. Save the antibacterial stuff for when you have a cut or other open wound that really requires disinfecting. The product will be much more effective because the bacteria haven't been able to "practice" against it.

387 **HOSPITAL SNOBBERY CAN BE OK** ■ Whenever you have the choice, pick a hospital that must compete for consumer health-care dollars. The best ER doctors in Mooseknuckle or even Cincinnati will not have seen as many cases of your problem

as their counterparts in Chicago or Los Angeles. At a small-town hospital that's the only game in town, you have the advantage of being known to the staff; but your own physician would also know you at a larger facility, and may have much more experience and resources to benefit you. It's not snobbery to choose the hospital that has the best reputation, it's smart strategizing.

388 **HOW COME THE EMERGENCY ROOM IS TAKING SO DARN LONG?** ■ As you sit and wait in the emergency room, keep repeating to yourself: "This is a good sign." After initial assessment, patient care is prioritized based on the nature of the illness or injury. Life-threatening, critical-care situations are always given top priority—and usually that order is shifting constantly as new, unexpected patients arrive. So if breathing or bleeding emergencies are ahead of you in line, it's a sort of blessing in disguise: You are in better shape than those folks. However, you have a right to ask about an estimated time for treatment.

389 **DON'T FLIP OUT IF THE WAITING ROOM IS FULL** ■ Don't panic if you arrive at the emergency room and find almost every chair filled. Not all of those people are actually ahead of you. Factors you never considered may affect how long it takes to receive treatment. A patient might need a specific room whose equipment is already in use. Procedures like X rays, lab tests, and scans take time to be processed, and patients and their families have to wait. Specialists may have to be consulted and have to examine a patient. And some people could be waiting for admission to the hospital. So just find yourself a chair—and don't panic until you have all the facts.

390 **BEAUTY AND DELIGHTFULNESS ARE GOOD ER STRATEGIES** ■ It's not fair, but it's true: Human beings respond better and more quickly to more attractive people. Since it's too late to pick better-looking ancestors, raise your attractiveness factor by being as delightful as possible to the ER staff. That doesn't mean being a doormat or sucking up, but it does mean being as polite and pleasant as you can manage—even when you're sick and scared. Be sure that anyone accompanying you is also polite, but direct. Of course the people most urgently in need of care will be seen first, but wouldn't it be great to go to the head of the line of everyone at your level of need? Be someone the staff won't cringe at, and your calls for a nurse may be (appropriately) prioritized.

391 THE ONE-TIME-ONLY NUCLEAR ATTENTION OPTION ■

Your real, sincere-but-not-considered-emergency calls for assistance or attention may be ignored by overworked staffers, or you may be left in a room with no one checking back on you after someone has downshifted your crisis. If you've been foresighted enough to put a whistle (even a cheap plastic coach's whistle will do) in your grab-and-go bag (see Tip No. 385) you will have a way to reach past the curtains and down the halls to alert a staffer.

Warning: this is for true emergencies only, to be used by people admitted alone, who have no one else to send or speak for them! You can do this only once—then you'll be considered obnoxious.

You'll also scare the heck out of cardiac patients on the next gurney, and you should expect your whistle to be confiscated after you've tooted it. But because nurse-call buttons sometimes don't work, and some ER staffers have been at their jobs so long that they forget there's a person with feelings attached to your paperwork, having a last-resort strategy to summon attention from a distance is as easy as forethought.

392 YOUR HEALTH-CARE PROXY I: EVERY PERSON WITH DIABETES NEEDS ONE ■

A health-care proxy is a legal document that you absolutely, positively must have just in case you are unable—even temporarily—to make treatment decisions for yourself. Laws vary from state to state. In some states, only your health-care agent—not a family member—has the authority to make these crucial decisions.

393 **YOUR HEALTH-CARE PROXY II: DECISIONS, DECISIONS** ■ As long as you are a competent adult over the age of eighteen, you can appoint a health-care agent (who also must be competent and over the age of eighteen) by signing a health-care proxy. You don't need a lawyer or a notary, just two adult witnesses, neither of whom can be your agent or alternate agent.

394 **YOUR HEALTH-CARE PROXY III: MAKE YOUR WISHES CLEAR** ■ You can and should indicate your specific orders on the proxy form, including your choice of life support if you are in a coma, treatment if you have a terminal illness, and whether you want artificial nutrition or hydration, and under what conditions.

If your agent does not know your wishes, he or she is legally required to act in your own best interest. However, you are much wiser to discuss your wishes in advance.

395 **YOUR HEALTH-CARE PROXY IV: WANT TO CHANGE THEM?** ■ Your proxy isn't written in stone. If you want to cancel it, change your health-care agent, or change any instructions, just fill out a new form.

You can also direct that this proxy expires on a specific date, or if certain events take place. Otherwise, your proxy will be valid indefinitely.

If you choose your spouse as your health-care agent or alternate and you become divorced or legally separated, the appointment is canceled automatically. If you want your former spouse to remain your agent, state this on your current form and date it or complete a new form naming him or her.

396 **YOUR HEALTH-CARE PROXY: MAKE SIX COPIES** ■ You need at least six copies of your health-care proxy. Deliver them to:

(1)   your health-care agent

(2)   your doctor (or doctors)

(3)   your attorney

(4)   at least one family member or close friend

And also:

(5)   keep one with all your other important papers—but not in your safe-deposit box because no one else may be able to get it.

(6)   keep one in your wallet next to your driver's license or insurance card, in case you have an accident and are admitted to the hospital, or even have outpatient surgery.

397 ALWAYS GET A SECOND OPINION BEFORE SURGERY OR TREATMENT FOR A SERIOUS CONDITION ■

Although fewer than one in four Americans gets a second opinion from another specialist, these visits are often covered by insurance. Second opinions can protect you if the first specialist made a diagnostic error or test results are not conclusive. If the specialist uses words like "We're *not sure*" or "You *seem*," get a second opinion.

Best bet: Consult a physician in a related field, like a gastroenterologist or an oncologist who does not do surgery. Make it clear that you are seeing this specialist for a second opinion only. (You can always change your mind and use him or her for longer-term care.)

398 SOMETIMES THIRD OPINIONS ARE NECESSARY ■ If the first two opinions disagree, you may need a third.

(In that case, many insurance companies and Medicare cover the third opinion.)

Get a clear consensus that the suggested treatment is the best one for you. Most conditions can wait a few weeks while you weigh all the options.

399 TRUST YOUR INSTINCTS ■ You are the world's greatest expert on your body, personality, and lifestyle. A treatment that is right for someone else may be wrong for you. Let your doctor's opinion guide your decision, but not overrule it.

400 DISCUSS ALTERNATIVE THERAPIES WITH YOUR PRIMARY CARE PROVIDER ■ Most medical groups are expanding into alternative medicine, and your primary physician is your best guide. Chiropractic, acupuncture, and physical therapy are usually covered and may help you.

401 VITAL SIGNS MAY NOT BE VITAL IN YOUR CASE ■ Ask your doctor whether your vital signs *really* need to be checked every four hours. (If not, you may be able to get a good night's rest.)

402 PERSONALIZE YOUR HOSPITAL SPACE ■ Brighten your little corner with flowers, photos of family and pets, and your kids' artwork. Not only will they cheer you up, they'll also send a message to the hospital staff that you are a real person, not just a chart.

403 YOUR VERY OWN DO NOT DISTURB SIGN ■ This advice comes directly from my internist:
Bring a Magic Marker, adhesive tape, and some paper with you. With your doctor's permission, make a DO NOT DISTURB sign and tape it on your door.

404 VISITORS INFLUENCE THE STAFF'S TREATMENT OF YOU ■ Have relatives and friends visit you in the hospital. The staff knows if you've never had visitors and may be inclined to pay less attention to you. Visitors will advocate for you and send the message that other people care about you.

405 **KNOW YOUR NUMBERS** ■ Before you leave for the hospital, jot down these numbers and keep them handy:

▶ your blood pressure
▶ your hemoglobin A1C and microalbumin

Asthmatics, know your peak flow. (You should be testing at home.) It lets the hospital choose the best treatment for you.

406 **AND YOUR OTHER TESTS** ■ Bring a copy of your most recent EKG, especially if you are at risk for cardiovascular disease. Your family doctor should have some scaled-down extra copies in your file. You may not know how to read your EKG, but the hospital staff will, and they will have something to use as a yardstick to compare with any new tests.

407 **ONE MORE THING TO BRING** ■ If you have glaucoma, bring your drops with you; my family doctor says that hospitals usually don't have them. However, some hospitals won't let you bring any drugs from home, so if there's time, check first, to see if that's the case.

408 **LEARN EVERYONE'S NAME** ■ When you address doctors and nurses by name, they know you know who they are and, technically it makes them responsible for any problems on their watch. Also, treating the staff like individuals rather than their job description gets you better care.

409 BEFORE YOU START TREATMENT ■ Ask your doctor about side effects, benefits and risks, and recommended reading, including reliable Web sites.

Bring a relative or friend with you for support and ask him or her to take notes for you, or bring a tape recorder so that you can replay the doctor's diagnosis and instructions as often as necessary.

410 GET EXPLANATIONS ■ Make your questions more palatable by saying, "I don't understand. Would you please explain that more simply?" And if you don't understand the medical terminology, as many patients don't, ask your doctor to define every word.

411 KNOW WHAT YOU'RE BEING GIVEN—AND WHY ■ Hospital "accidents" happen. Minimize the risk that they happen to you. Know the pills and other treatments that the nurses and technicians give you. Ask them these questions:

Who are you? (name and job title)
What is this?
Who ordered this? Why? What's it supposed to do?
Are you trained to administer this? (Sometimes nurses and technicians cover for each other.)

412 MAKE SURE THEY WASH THEIR HANDS BEFORE THEY TOUCH YOU ■ The statistics are terrifying: Nearly 90,000 Americans die each year from infections they acquired as hospital patients. According to data reported in the October 2003 issue of the *Journal of the American Medical Association*, hospital-acquired infections were responsible for more than nine extra days in the hospital, on average. The worst infections—postsurgical sepsis in the bloodstream—resulted in much longer stays and a 22 percent increased risk of death.

One simple move can minimize your risk: Say to any staffer who comes near you, "I'm afraid of hospital infections." If they don't take the hint, be blunt: "Please wash your hands."

413 **KEEP YOUR DIGNITY IN THE HOSPITAL** ■ No one said you had to wear hospital-issue johnnies, those unpleasant short gowns that are open all the way up the back. Wearing them is uncomfortable, embarrassing, and dehumanizing. Bring your own PJs, robe, underwear, and slippers. Men, your favorite T-shirt and briefs or boxers are fine. And women, your favorite sexy nightgown can cheer you up. Express your individuality—your self-esteem really needs it now!

414 **CHECK YOUR SURGEON'S AND ANESTHESIOLOGIST'S TRACK RECORD** ■ Make sure that your surgeon and anesthesiologist don't have an ugly record of malpractice suits. States vary in making this information available to ordinary people, but doctors or lawyers can access it easily. Your best bet is to ask your family doctor or another doctor you trust about these specialists' track record.

415 **HAVE A PRESURGERY DISCUSSION WITH YOUR ANESTHESIOLOGIST** ■ Several days before your surgery, ask your anesthesiologist these questions:

What drug will you use?
Is it all right to use with the drugs I am taking? Go through your list.
How is it administered?
Why did you select it?
Is it recommended for people with diabetes?
What are the risks? The side effects?

It may sound paranoid, but it's a smart way to protect yourself.

416 TRY FOR AN EARLY RELEASE . . . ■ Sounds like prison, doesn't it? But home healing is usually better and faster. Many medical treatments can be continued at your home, and there's much less risk of infection.

417 . . . BUT FIGHT PREMATURE DISCHARGE ■ If you can't keep food or liquid down, can't go to the bathroom without help, have pain that can't be controlled by pills, or feel disoriented or unsteady, you are not ready to go home.

If the hospital still tries to discharge you, insist on talking to your doctor. If your doctor can't get your stay extended, talk to the discharge planner or patient advocate.

Go up the ladder. Your next step is contacting your insurance carrier and the hospital administrator. If you are on Medicare, hospitals must give you a toll-free number to call to appeal their decisions.

418 "PLEASE AUTOGRAPH MY LEG" ■ Surgeons operating on the wrong side of the body are grist for the newspapers. These blunders are rare, but they happen often enough that the American Academy of Orthopaedic Surgeons has advised its members to initial the surgery site beforehand. Ask your surgeon to mark the site and initial it—in case of trouble, this has more legal standing than your marking the area with lipstick.

419 BE THE SECOND OR THIRD SURGERY IN THE MORNING ■ During the first surgery of the day, the surgeon and the surgical team are often still warming up, not quite at peak performance. The second or third slot is much better, and you'll still get your immediate postoperative care during the day shift, when the nursing staff is at full strength.

420 **GET WALKING ASAP** ■ Walking as soon as possible reduces the risk of developing dangerous blood clots in your legs. If you need support, ask a nurse, friend, or relative to lend an arm. And ask for special elastic stockings while you are recovering if you are overweight or have varicose veins.

421 **PREVENT DEEP-VEIN THROMBOSIS (DVT)** ■ Deep-vein thrombosis (DVT) refers to blood clots that develop in the legs, often as a result of immobility in bed. But they can travel up to the lungs (pulmonary emboli) and become potentially fatal for up to eight weeks after surgery.

Ask your doctor what is being done to prevent DVT; compression stockings and blood thinners are often prescribed.

Warning signs: Leg pain or redness, problems breathing. *Call your doctor immediately.*

422 **KNOW WHO'S IN CHARGE** ■ Several specialists may examine you while you're in the hospital. Make sure that one doctor coordinates your treatment so that the chance of over-lapping or conflicting orders is minimized. Ideally, your primary-care physician or a colleague should visit you every day.

After your body, your wallet is at greatest risk in a hospital. Imagine being billed $129 for a "mucus recovery system"! Believe it or not, that was hospitalspeak for a box of tissues! One middle-aged man, in for hip surgery, was charged for a crib and newborn blood tests!

Estimates on hospital overcharges run up to $10 billion a year, with an average of $1,300 per hospital stay. Many experts believe that many of these charges are deliberate. Here are some tips you can use to pre-vent your getting clipped and having your credit destroyed:

423 **AVOID HOSPITAL OVERCHARGES I: KNOW WHAT'S COVERED** ■ If it's not an emergency, check your insurance policy to find out exactly what it will cover and how much it will pay. Read the "Exceptions and Exclusions" section over and over because it spells out what your policy will *not* cover.

424 **AVOID HOSPITAL OVERCHARGES II: ALL ABOUT ROOM CHARGES** ■ Call the hospital's billing department and find out exactly what the room charges cover. Better yet, ask them to fax you a list. You may need this ammunition. If they're charging you for soap and a toothbrush, bring your own.

425 **AVOID HOSPITAL OVERCHARGES III: YOUR DOCTOR CAN HELP** ■ Ask your doctor about how much your treatment will cost and whether you can bring and use your own prescription drugs to avoid paying for the hospital's medication.

426 **AVOID HOSPITAL OVERCHARGES IV: CHECK THE OTHER DOCTORS** ■ Make sure that *all* the doctors who will be treating you—the anesthesiologist, the surgeon, the pathologist, the rehabilitation specialist—participate in your insurance plan. If not, your charges may be astronomical!

427 **AVOID HOSPITAL OVERCHARGES V: KEEP TRACK** ■ Keep a record of medications, tests, and treatments, or ask a relative or friend to do it for you.

428 **AVOID HOSPITAL OVERCHARGES VI: DON'T PAY THE BILL YET** ■ Regardless of what the staff tells you, never pay your bill before you leave the hospital.

429 **AVOID HOSPITAL OVERCHARGES VII: GET AN ITEMIZED BILL** ■ Compare the bill to your record of treatment. Read it very, very carefully. If anything looks vague, demand an itemized bill—every state requires hospitals to do so.

Ask for your medical records, too, and compare then with the bill to check whether or not you received the medications and treatments you have been billed for.

430 AVOID HOSPITAL OVERCHARGES VIII: GO TO THE TOP ■ Hospital billing departments hope that you will cave in and pay unquestioningly. *Don't.* Write to the hospital administrator, then the hospital president and—if necessary—every single individual on their board of trustees. (You can find their names on the hospital's Web site). These people all know that bad publicity can cost them big bucks in contributions.

431 CALL IN THE CAVALRY ■ You have some powerful watchdog organizations on your side. If the hospital stonewalls you or threatens to ruin your credit, try these, and be firm:

American Hospital Association (your state's chapter or the national organization)
National Health Care Anti-Fraud Association
Blue Cross/Blue Shield Division of Special Investigations

5

Exercise

432 **JUST DON'T CALL IT EXERCISE** ■ Many of us have a hatred of exercise that dates back to grade school, when we were the chubby, slow, ungraceful kids who were always chosen last on teams.

Nevertheless, physical activity is a crucial component of good diabetes care. There's a simple solution. Find something you like to do. Stroll through city streets and parks. Wander through museums or malls with a friend. Go for a bike ride or play volleyball with your kids or grandkids. Go out dancing or put on some music and dance at home.

Just don't call it exercise!

433 **SUCCESSFUL PROGRAMS START SLOWLY** ■ Start very slowly. If you're out of shape, start with a five- or ten-minute walk. You can even walk around your house—set a kitchen timer.

Try lighter weights: three- or five-pound dumbbells.

The winning strategy? Feeling "Hey, this isn't so bad; I can stick with this." Or maybe even "I feel good; I'll do a little more of this tomorrow."

434 **DOUBLE DUTY FOR DOGWALKERS** ■ Get an extra workout when you walk your dog. Keep the leash short and step away from it until you can feel the pull. Bend over slowly until your head is in line with your waist, forming a right angle with your legs. Then straighten up slowly. Repeat four or five times, then move on and bend again.

435 **WALK AROUND IN CIRCLES** ■ This tip works well for city dwellers.

Do you enjoy walking, but hate being stopped by traffic lights? You won't lose momentum if you go around the block. In most cities, three circuits measures a little over one mile.

Increase your workout by finding a block with one uphill and one downhill side.

436 **REWARD YOURSELF!** ■ Motivate yourself to walk or bike instead of taking public transport by banking your carfare. Put the money in a clear glass jar or bowl so that seeing it will inspire you to add to the kitty.

When the container is full—or every month or so—reward yourself with a little treat and start the cycle again. Pedicures are an appropriate indulgence and are enjoyed by men as much as by women.

437 **REORGANIZE YOUR KITCHEN** ■ Make your kitchen *less* convenient to get more of a workout you don't have to think about.

Put things you use every day—like coffee filters, sugar substitutes, your most-used pots and pans—on the highest and lowest shelves. If you need to bend, stretch, or climb on a step stool several times a day, you're exercising without realizing it.

438 **"SOFT" EXERCISE WORKS!** ■ You probably know that exercise reduces your risk of cardiovascular disease by 30 percent. But did you know that your workout doesn't have to be hard? Brisk walking for 30 minutes at least five days a week will give you the same reduction in risk as more vigorous exercise like running, with less wear and tear on your hips, knees, and ankles.

439 **USE A BED OR A CHAIR** ■ Is it difficult for you to move around? You can do many exercises lying in bed or sitting in a chair. As your body becomes more flexible and you develop more energy, increase the number of repetitions you do and the length of your workout sessions.

440 **LET THE WATER HELP YOU EXERCISE** ■ Many over-weight people excel at swimming because their bodies are naturally buoyant and they don't have to fight gravity. Their knees, hips, and ankles don't hurt as much, either.

If swimming laps bore you, try a water aerobics class, or do the exercises alone.

441 **GYM MEMBERSHIPS ARE TAX-DEDUCTIBLE** ■ You can deduct the cost of your gym membership and of any exercise classes as a medical expense on your federal and local income-tax returns.

Get a letter from your doctor stating that the gym membership and classes are necessary for weight loss and diabetes care, and attach copies of the letter to your tax returns.

442 **TRY BEFORE YOU BUY** ■ Human nature being what it is, we all start off with the best of intentions. We'll buy exercise equipment—also tax-deductible with a doctor's letter—and use it faithfully, or join a gym and go faithfully.

But then reality or inertia intrude, and that exercise equipment becomes an expensive clothes rack and the gym membership becomes just another card in your wallet.

Save your money! Try a one-month membership at the gym, or a one-month rental of that jazzy exercise machine. See how often you use them before you buy them.

443 FIDGET! ■ Make use of spare minutes and rev up your metabolism without thinking about it. All of these count as exercise:

Waiting for the elevator? Do heel or toe raises or contract your glutes.
Watching the clock in a waiting room? Sit up straight in your chair, raise your legs, and do leg extensions.
Waiting to cross the street? March or jog in place.

444 STOP USING THE REMOTE CONTROL ■ Move around the room. At least, get up to change the TV program. Movement is cumulative. Don't be a couch potato!

445 TAKING YOUR DOCTOR'S ADVICE ■ You have often heard that you should consult a physician before undertaking any exercise program. *However*, make sure that you ask your doctor what he/she knows about that particular form of exercise.

446 TRY WEIGHT TRAINING ■ Weight training builds lean muscle mass. That speeds up your metabolic rate, which helps burn fat and carbohydrates.

Some forms of weight training can be hard on your joints. The best system is Super Slow, which requires fewer repetitions to achieve the same results, while not putting so much stress on the joints.

447 ADVANTAGES OF YOGA, TAI CHI, AND QI GONG ■ Yoga, tai chi, and qi gong emphasize flexibility and build stamina and endurance. You work slowly, which helps older, sedentary people with diabetes. All three systems are designed to open up the flow of chi (life energy) and to improve breathing, which oxygenates the blood and increases circulation and metabolism.

448 MARTIAL ARTS STRESSES DIFFERENT PARTS OF YOUR BODY ■ Which part of your body will vary from style to style. Punching and kicking forms place more stress on your ankles, knees, hips, wrists, and shoulders. Throwing and grappling will stress your hips.

449 YOUR MARTIAL-ARTS CLASS MAY NOT BE VERY AEROBIC ■ Many martial-arts programs aren't. If your class emphasizes learning techniques, you can spend a lot of time waiting your turn to perform the action. "Martial arts" is about combat and, like combat, can often mean long periods of waiting, followed by short bursts of intense activity.

450 BLACK BELT? RED FLAG! ■ Avoid any school that *guarantees* you a black belt or wants you to commit to a long-term contract. Ask to watch a class or two to get some idea of the activity and of the teacher's ability. If you are refused, go elsewhere. If you are told that the techniques are "too dangerous for the casual or uncommitted observer," run—do not walk—to the nearest exit!

451 TAKE ADVANTAGE OF VIDEOS ■ OK, you don't have the time or money to go to a gym. Or your body embarrasses you.

You still have hundreds of choices. There are many exercise programs available. Borrow them from the library or rent them from the video store before you buy them.

452 BALLET ISN'T ONLY FOR KIDS ■ Ballet classes work well for adults. Beginners' ballet emphasizes balance and coordination and develops flexibility, grace, and posture. Take a class at your local Y, or try videos.

453 TRY BELLY DANCING ■ Here is an exercise where generous curves are a distinct advantage. You can be overweight and still feel very sensual, which should motivate you to continue this sexy, satisfying exercise.

454 VARY YOUR EXERCISE ROUTINE ■ Boredom is the enemy of self-discipline. We get tired of the workout routine, and soon we just quit.

Fight the inevitable monotony by varying your exercise routine. Racewalk one day, climb stairs another, go swimming or dancing later in the week. Variety will keep your interest sparked.

455 PILATES WITHOUT THE MACHINE ■ The Pilates system offers its disciples long, lean, beautifully toned muscles—strong, but not bulging. But Pilates machines cost hundreds of dollars and occupy lots of space.

Some excellent Pilates programs now available on videotape are designed to be used without the machines. Instead, you do the low-impact exercises on the floor very, very slowly, so that you get the gain without the pain.

456 HAVE A BAD-WEATHER ALTERNATIVE ■ Don't let rain or snow dampen your plans. Find an indoor exercise alternative for nasty weather. Some of the best for combining pleasure with exercise are mall walking and visiting museums.

457 GET A PEDOMETER ■ This lightweight little gadget can inspire you just by clocking how much walking you do every day. Every step counts, whether it's housework, doing errands, or racewalking.

If you need encouragement, keep track of your weekly distances and try to increase them every week or every other week. Or calculate the distance from your home to some marvelous destination—New York? San Francisco? London? Paris? Samarkand? the length of Hadrian's Wall?—and log how long it takes you to get there. Keep a map and a Magic Marker stuck to the fridge!

Before you buy your pedometer, make sure that it will not stop counting if you stop moving for more than fifteen minutes, and make sure that you can return or exchange it within two weeks if you find that it is inaccurate.

458 PROCRASTINATING DOESN'T PAY OFF ■ "Tomorrow and tomorrow" isn't just the beginning of a *Macbeth* soliloquy; it sums up many people's attitude to exercise. Starting your exercise plan "tomorrow" *is* great, but when the sun rises, tomorrow becomes today, and somehow your plan never gets off the drawing board.

459 THE DELIGHTS OF DANCING ■ Dancing is a feel-good, total-body exercise. Many forms are good for a lifetime: ballroom or freestyle, folk dancing, English or Scottish country dancing, salsa, and line or square dancing. The best part is that the level of participation is up to you. Some forms are strenuous; the country dance "Strip the Willow" is best reserved for Iron Man competitors.

Many kinds of dance do not require partners, a blessing for single people, and many types of dance have clubs in many U.S. cities.

Note: If you are interested in ballroom dancing, avoid taking lessons at the big dance-school chains, and especially of being "persuaded" to sign expensive yearlong—or even "lifetime" contracts.

460 EASY RIDER ■ Back problems? Knees or hips painful? You can still get the exercise benefits of bicycle riding. Try a recumbent bike. This exercise machine lets you lie comfortably on your back and pedal away. You get a minimal-impact workout that improves your circulation and burns calories without stressing your joints.

461 BROOMSTICK TRICK ■ You can use a household broom or mop as an exercise tool. Wrap your fingers around the ends of the stick and turn to the right as far as you can comfortably. Then turn to the left. The stick provides a little weight and momentum, so you'll get more of a workout. This exercise is a wonderful waist-whittler.

462 HOUSECLEANING COUNTS AS EXERCISE ■ Think of all the bending, stretching, and reaching you do when you dust, sweep, vacuum, and scrub. You may not think of this as exercise, but it is. An hour of heavy housecleaning will burn as many calories as an hour of racewalking. (You may want to check your blood glucose afterward.)

463 GARDENING DOES, TOO ■ You dig, plant, water, prune, harvest. It's a very pleasant aerobic workout. And being out in the sun gives you vitamin D, necessary for building and protecting your bones. (But please wear a sunblock.)

464 PACE! ■ Your cordless or cell phone can help you exercise. Don't just sit there when you're talking, pace up and down. You'll get some exercise without realizing it.

465 LENGTHEN YOUR STRIDE ■ To increase benefits from exercising, lengthen your stride when you walk. Just lengthening it by 5" or 6" will do the trick. Your posture will improve, too!

466 PERK UP YOUR WORKOUT ■ If you like your morning coffee, exercising in the morning could give your workout a boost.

In a recent study, people who consumed about a coffee cup's worth of caffeine before their workouts experienced less exercise-caused muscle pain during their exertions. Researchers speculate that the caffeine could boost exercise endurance.

467 BED EXERCISE I: LEG RAISES ■ Lying in bed, raise one leg slowly as high as you can, toes pointed, to a count of ten. Hold for a count of ten, then lower to a count of ten. Then do the same with the other leg. Alternate sides and do five raises each side, increasing the number of leg raises gradually. Keep on increasing the number of leg raises until it just begins to hurt. That's when the effect is greatest.

468 BED EXERCISE II: HIP ROLLS ■ Lying on your back, swing one leg across your body as far as possible without lifting your hips off the mattress, to a count of five. Hold for a count of five, then swing your leg back to a count of five. Repeat this sequence five times, then switch legs. Work up to five sets of ten leg swings on each side. (This is a wonderful waist whittler.)

469 BED EXERCISE III: BACK STRETCH ■ Lying on your back, pull your knees up to your chest. Hold for a count of five. Straighten your legs out and lower them to a count of ten. Using this slow count, repeat this movement until you cannot complete one.

As you get more flexible, make this exercise harder by extending your legs over your head and rolling up on your shoulders, then swinging them downward in a long arc to a count of ten. When you can do the whole exercise as a unit, you will stretch your back, tighten your abs, and strengthen your lower back all in one exercise. Gradually increase the number of repetitions, and also lengthen the count for each part.

470 **OFFICE EXERCISE: DESK CHECK** ■ For all exercises at your desk, be sure that your desk is either heavy enough or anchored well enough that you won't move it or tip it over. Be sure that your chair is stable, too.

471 **OFFICE EXERCISE I: PUSH-PULL** ■ This exercise requires a chair with wheels. At your desk, raise your feet slightly off the floor. Use your arms to pull yourself forward, then push backward as far as you can go. If you have room, lean forward as far as possible on the push and try to come to a full upright position on the pull.

472 **OFFICE EXERCISE II: LEG RAISES** ■ At your desk, raise your legs until they are completely extended straight out in front of you, then lower them. Use the same count as for the leg raises in bed. Grip the seat of your chair with your hands at your sides so that you can't use them to help raise your legs.

473 **OFFICE EXERCISE III: GLUTEUS CRUNCHES** ■ At your desk, extend your legs slightly off the floor. Raise them by clenching your buttocks. Use a count of five to raise, five to hold, and five to lower. Start with a set of five and increase gradually.

474 OFFICE EXERCISE IV: SHOULDER ROLLS ■ This exercise is less strenuous than the following one, so always do it first to warm up. Roll your shoulders backward slowly eight times, then forward slowly eight times. Do four or five sets.

This exercise will relieve back and neck strain that frequently accompanies heavy keyboard use, whether computer or musical.

475 OFFICE EXERCISE V: SHOULDER CIRCLES ■ With your arms fully extended, make small circles in the air so that your fingertips are moving only a few inches. Circle forward for a count of ten, hold for a count of ten, and then circle backward for a count of ten. Start with a set of five and increase gradually.

476 MAKE ISOMETRICS WORK FOR YOU ■ Isometrics is the exercise technique that pits one set of your body's muscles against their opposites. For example, put the heels of your hands together in front of your chest. Try to push one hand toward its opposite side, then reverse. You can also do this exercise with your hands placed over your head. Any way you can work your body's muscles against themselves will increase their strength and, if done long enough and with increasing effort, will help build muscle and increase your metabolism.

477 SORENESS = SUCCESS ■ Muscle growth is the result of muscle fiber being stretched and torn so that new muscle fiber grows in. Small wonder that your muscles are sore after a really hard workout, or that most exercise experts advise resting for a day between workouts.

If you feel sore, reward yourself with a long soak in a hot tub. Epsom salts and other mineral treatments help!

478 MUSIC, MAESTRO ∎ Did you know that orchestra conductors are extraordinarily long-lived? Their secret? The wonderful cardiovascular workout they get by moving their arms for hours nearly every day.

You'll get a great workout by playing conductor to symphonic music or operas for at least twenty minutes at a time.

479 LIGHTEN UP ∎ Light weights work well for beginning exercisers. You can find them right in your pantry. Cans of soup weighing approximately one pound are easy to wrap your fingers around. When you can do forty or fifty repetitions of two or three different exercises, it's time to move up to heavier weights.

Note: Anyone with retinopathy or high blood pressure should be very careful about lifting weights. Ask your doctor first!

480 BE INEFFICIENT ∎ Carry your packages and bags of groceries from your car one by one, to make as many trips as possible. This is an upper-body exercise that doesn't require any planning or thinking.

481 ADD WALKING TO YOUR DRIVING AND RIDING ∎ Take a more distant parking space and walk a little more. Make this part of your daily routine. If you use public transportation, get off a few stops before your usual one and walk to your destination.

482 TAKE ADVANTAGE OF TV COMMERCIAL BREAKS ∎ Don't just sit there or make a beeline for snacks. Walk in place (or run!), do push-ups against the nearest wall, or do knee bends.

You'll find that you're exercising for at least ten minutes every hour!

483 STAIRWAY TO SUCCESS ■ If you work in an office building or live in an apartment building, you can *be* a stair climber rather than using one at the health club. Start by walking up or down only one flight each time instead of using the elevator for the whole trip. Increase your stair climbing by one flight up and one flight down every week. Make sure that you climb up *and* down because you use different sets of muscles for each exercise. Soon you'll be zipping up and down the stairs, avoiding the elevator crush, and giving yourself a wonderful cardiovascular workout.

484 TAKE A WALK AFTER DINNER ■ Going for a walk after dinner offers many benefits:

▶ It removes you from the kitchen and dining room, which may tempt you to eat more.
▶ It revs up your metabolism when you need it most.
▶ It's a great stress and tension reliever.
▶ It can give you and your partner and/or your kids some uninterrupted time together.

485 LIGHT WEIGHTS BOOST STRETCHING ■ Grabbing a set of light weights could help improve your range of motion.

Stretching is a great way to improve your flexibility and balance and increase your range of motion. Research suggest that stretching with a set of light weights in your hands may bring even better results. Stick to very light weights—one pound or less—until you become accustomed to the added load.

486 PLAY A MUSICAL INSTRUMENT ■ Yes, this counts as exercise, too. Playing most musical instruments gives you a powerful aerobic payoff. Think of the deep-breathing exercise you get in playing a wind instrument or brass, or the powerful upper-body workout you get in playing the piano, drums, or a string instrument.

487 FLOOR PLAY ■ Sit on the floor with your legs spread, back straight. Play jacks or pick-up sticks alone or with a friend. Pick up marbles of different sizes with your toes. Have fun!

488 KEEP YOUR EQUIPMENT HANDY ■ When you have to plow through your closets to find your exercise gear, you're less likely to use it consistently. Keep your outfit and equipment in one accessible place so that you'll use it often.

489 YOU CAN HANDLE IT ■ If you can't touch your toes or have other problems with flexibility, use the handles on chests of drawers or kitchen cabinets to reach lower and lower. These heavy pieces of furniture are very stable and won't move as you reach down farther and farther.

490 MAKE AN INVESTMENT IN YOUR FITNESS ■ Think of fitness as a long-term investment in your life, just like any kind of financial retirement plan. Just as you put away money in a 401(k) or IRA every year in order to benefit from it years from now, keep your body moving over the long term will pay off when you are much older.

Why is this important? According to the National Center for Health Statistics, a person who lives to age 65 will live, on average, 17.9 more years. Experts say that even slow, low-impact fitness programs can make your biological age 10 years younger than your chronological age.

491 DO THE FLAMINGO ■ No, it's not a close relative of the Funky Chicken. It's an exercise designed to strengthen your ankles and improve your balance so that you are less likely to take a nasty fall as you get older.

I've named this exercise for its appearance. Warning: It's harder than it looks, but the results and protection it will give you are worth the effort.

Stand in a doorway where the floor has no sill and is absolutely flat. Place your palms on either side of the doorway a little below shoulder height for balance. Now stand on one leg and raise the other, knee bent. Hold this position as long as you can; then reverse legs.

At first you may be able to hold the position for only two or three minutes on each side. Work up to five or six if you can.

When this exercise becomes too easy, stop using your hands for balance and keep them at your sides.

492 **SPEND ONE HOUR WITH A PRO** ■ Just one hour with a personal trainer can be the best investment you make in your exercise routine. In that hour, your trainer should be able to diagnose the areas of your body that need work, teach you the best exercises to achieve the desired results, and the most effective order to do them.

To find a qualified trainer, check these professional groups on the Internet: American College of Sports Medicine, American Council on Exercise, and the National Strength and Conditioning Association. Then phone the trainers themselves and check at least three of their recent references.

493 **POINTED ADVICE** ■ Increase the benefits from your leg exercises by alternately pointing and flexing your toes. This movement will stretch your hamstrings and help build up your calf muscles (gastrocnemius) and the muscle that lies along your shin (soleus).

494 **TRY A TREADMILL HIGH** ■ Hitting the treadmill can give you an amphetaminelike lift that lasts for twenty-

four hours. British researchers found that people who run on a treadmill for thirty minutes produced almost twice as much phenylethylamine, a brain chemical similar to amphetamine, than people who were couch potatoes.

495 **YOUR VERY OWN BALLET BARRE** ■ Improvise an at-home ballet barre for doing forward and backward leg lifts. You won't have to do any work or move any furniture.

Although chairs are often recommended for holding on to, they are too lightweight and can slide across the floor, creating a potential hazard. Instead, use the top of your bedroom dresser, which is heavy enough to provide good support.

As a bonus, dressers often have mirrors that you can use to check the posture of your upper body while you do the leg lifts.

496 **COMBINE CARDIOVASCULAR AND RESISTANCE EXERCISES** ■ You'll get more "bang" for your "exercise buck" and save time with exercise that combines cardiovascular workouts with resistance training. Some of the best: riding your bike, doing step aerobics, and walking or jogging up and down hills.

497 **STRETCH AT THE END, TOO** ■ Most people do stretches for warm-ups, before they work out. But stretching at the end of a workout has its own benefits. Stretching when your muscles are warm enhances your flexibility more than stretches at the beginning of your workout, when your muscles are still cold.

498 **STAY FLEXIBLE: UPPER BODY** ■ Stretching your triceps aids upper-body flexibility. Place a bath towel along your back. Hold the top in your right hand and grasp the bottom in your left hand. Climb up the towel with your left hand as high as you can reach. Alternate hands and repeat.

499

STAY FLEXIBLE: LOWER BODY ■ Stretch the muscles in your lower leg by placing your hands against a wall, elbows straight and arms extended. Bend your right knee and step back one to two feet with your left leg, foot flat on the floor. Hold. Then alternate legs. Do this exercise five times.

500

THE 10,000-STEP PRESCRIPTION ■ Exercise gurus urge us to walk at least 10,000 steps every day. This number translates as approximately 4.5 miles (1 step = approximately 28.5 inches), but remember: Every step counts.

You may want to start by getting some baseline figures. Use a pedometer on two weekdays plus one weekend day, total the mileage, and divide by 3 to get your average daily distance in miles. You can then convert this figure to steps, if you like, by multiplying it by 2,200.

If you discover that you are walking only about 2 miles a day, increase your walking slowly, adding 200–300 steps a day.

501

FIND YOUR BEST STRIDE BY IGNORING IT ■ Maybe you *don't* need to change your walking or running stride. Your doing "what comes naturally" is safer than consciously changing your stride, which can stress your muscles and joints, thus raising the risk of injury.

502

LIFTING WEIGHTS BANISHES BELLY FAT ■ Belly fat is dangerous. It increases the risk of diabetes and cardiovascular disease. Over a period of a few months, lifting light weights for multiple repetitions replaces fat with muscle, builds endurance, and reduces the risk of these deadly diseases.

503

BE A SILVER STAR ■ Silver Sneakers classes, offered at many Ys and health clubs, are designed specifically for older exercisers who may have arthritis or other problems. The aerobic and strength exercises are paced gently but effectively for people over fifty-five.

504 **SLOWER WALKING WORKS!** ■ Just getting out there is good for you, and it turns out that it's not the speed, but the distance that burns calories and pounds. Think of the tortoise and the hare, smile, and keep on walking.

505 **WHERE WALKERS BEAT RUNNERS** ■ Surprise! Walkers actually beat runners. New research finds that while both running and walking boost your energy and mood in as little as fifteen minutes, only walkers report feeling better *during* those fifteen minutes. Feeling good while you walk—rather than just afterward—helps encourage continuing activity.

506 **ESCALATOR STRATEGY: WALK WHILE YOU RIDE** ■ You can get more of a workout by walking up the escalator than climbing a flight of stairs. That's because the treads on escalators are so much higher. Walking up the escalator burns seven times more calories than standing still, and you'll get to your floor in only half the time.

507 **GO MALL WALKING** ■ Warm, light, and safe in the winter, cool in the summer, malls beat running tracks hands down. Whether you join a group or go it alone, mall walking offers a pleasant way to exercise, and you can judge your progress by how far around the mall you can go.

508 **DON'T RESIST RESISTANCE BANDS** ■ Resistance bands are lightweight rubber strips, inexpensive, portable, but strong enough to give you a good workout. Exercise guru Denise Austin uses them in many powerful exercises that work the upper and lower body muscles simultaneously, a blessing for the time-challenged.

509 DO IT IN THE MOONLIGHT ■ Summer evenings are an ideal time for exercising. The temperature has cooled down, and racewalking and running are much more comfortable.

Take advantage of this special time of lingering twilights to take longer-than-usual walks with your partner, family, or friends. Make plans for barbecues, picnics, and parties.

510 YOGA MAY FIGHT SERIOUS DISEASE ■ Besides boosting strength and flexibility and helping you relax and feel good, yoga may actually ward off disease.

Researchers at the Cleveland Clinic Foundation found that practicing yoga for as little as one month reduced the need for pain medication in people with arthritis, chronic back pain, and carpal tunnel syndrome.

Other studies found that yoga reduced the number of angina attacks in people with cardiovascular disease and that yoga may help control high blood pressure as effectively as some medications. Through its breathing exercises, yoga may also reduce the severity of chronic bronchitis and asthma.

511 THE EXERCISE OF LAUGHTER ■ Researchers at Stanford University have found that laughing for thirty seconds produces the same aerobic benefits as working out for three minutes on a rowing machine. What a pleasant way to strengthen your abdominals! Bring on those classic *Looney Tunes* cartoons, *Johnny Bravo*, and *The Kids in the 'Hood*.

512 JUMP TO IT! ■ Jumping rope offers great aerobic benefits while it builds flexibility and coordination and strengthens ankles and knees. One of its advantages is that it can be done indoors in limited space as well as outdoors. For extra fun, organize a jump-rope game with neighbors both older and younger than yourself. See how many of the schoolyard rope games and jump-rope rhymes you remember.

Get a game of double Dutch going. You'll really glow! Pass these routines on to your kids for wonderful multigenerational fun.

513

PICKUP GAMES ■ Who says that playgrounds and dead-end streets are only for kids? They can be ideal for casual sports games with loose rules, a chance for adults to put together softball or basketball games, to challenge their kids or the neighbors down the block.

If possible, try volleyball. If you can't locate or improvise a net, draw posts and a line representing the net in colored chalk. Volleyball is an excellent sport because players are in motion most of the time, combining lots of aerobics and stretching.

514

EXERCISE WHILE YOU FLY ■ Long periods of sitting still can be very risky, especially for people who have circulatory or cardiovascular problems. The culprit is deep vein thrombosis (DVT), the formation of blood clots in the legs. If a clot breaks free and travels to the heart or the lungs, it can be fatal.

Here are some exercises you can do in your seat to increase circulation and decrease the risk of DVT:

515

AIRBORNE I: ANKLE CIRCLES ■ Raise both feet off the floor. Rotate both of them simultaneously, making five circles toward the outside, then five toward the inside. Repeat this set five times.

516

AIRBORNE II: FOOT PUMPS ■ Rock back on your heels, raising your toes as far as possible. Hold for a count of ten, then lower them to the floor. Now rock onto your toes, raising your heels as far as possible. Hold for a count of ten, then lower them to the floor. Repeat five times.

517 **AIRBORNE III: SHOULDER ROLLS** ■ Place your arms on the armrests and move your shoulders in a circle from front to back ten times. Repeat from back to front ten times.

518 **AIRBORNE IV: KNEE-TO-CHEST STRETCHES** ■ Lean forward slightly and clasp your hands around one knee. Pull it slowly toward your chest and hold for fifteen seconds. Release. Switch to your other knee. Repeat five times.

519 **AIRBORNE V: SHOULDER STRETCHES** ■ Place your right hand on top of your left shoulder. Grasp your right elbow in your left hand and stretch your right shoulder gently toward your left side. Hold for fifteen seconds. Switch sides and repeat. Do this set five times.

520 **AIRBORNE VI: NECK ROLLS** ■ Relax your head and shoulders. Stretch your neck toward your left shoulder, hold for five seconds, roll your head slowly toward your chest, and then stretch toward your right shoulder. Hold for five seconds, then reverse, rolling your head from right to left. Repeat five times.

521 **EXERCISE PROTECTS YOUR BRAIN** ■ Exercise really prevents the loss of brain tissue and the accompanying memory loss that starts in our thirties. MRI studies show that poorly controlled blood-glucose levels cause the brain's key memory center (hippocampus) to shrink. But weight training, which builds muscle, regulates blood-glucose levels and helps prevent shrinkage of the brain tissue. Researchers believe that it can prevent or possibly even reverse memory loss.

522 **BE REFLECTIVE** ■ Play it safe when you exercise out-doors at dusk or night. Heighten your visibility to others by wearing reflective clothing, *not* clothing with reflective stripes, which reveal only a cartoonish outline of your shape.

523 **TAKE FITNESS WITH YOU I: CHOOSE HOTELS WITH EXERCISE FACILITIES** ■ Having a heavy travel sched-ule should not prevent your being able to work out. When you shop for a hotel, find out whether it has a gym, health club, pool—and whether there is a charge for using them. (If you get "sticker shock," find out if there is a running/walking trail near the hotel.)

524 **TAKE FITNESS WITH YOU II: USE THE PASSPORT PROGRAM** ■ Check whether the health club you belong to—or are thinking of joining—is one of the 4,000 clubs that participate in the International Health, Racquet & Sports Club Association (IHRSA) Passport Program, which lets you work out at any of the participating clubs while traveling in many countries around the world.

To use the Passport Program, log on to www.healthclubs.com, click Passport Program, and follow the instructions and the thumb-up icon. You'll be able to use any club more than fifty miles from your home club by paying a discounted guest fee. Call the guest club first to check hours, guest fee, and any restrictions.

525 **REV UP YOUR WALKING** ■ Perk up your walking workout by doing your usual warming up and stretching, then walking briskly for ten minutes, and then adding this quick little routine:

March in place for thirty seconds, lifting your knees high and swing-ing your arms. Walk briskly for one minute, then march in place again for thirty seconds. Continue walking briskly for ten minutes, then add a second little routine:

Skip for thirty seconds, swinging your arms, walk briskly for one minute, then skip for thirty seconds.

Now continue your walking routine.

526 HOOP IT UP! ■ Swinging a hula hoop around your middle can whittle your waistline and abs, trimming dangerous abdominal fat. It's a great cardiovascular workout, too.

Just make sure to rotate the hoop equally clockwise and counterclockwise. We tend to favor our stronger side, but you want to keep this workout evenly balanced.

527 MIND OVER MATTRESS ■ Drag your old mattress down to the basement or out to the backyard. Use it as a cushiony exercise mat or jump on it like a trampoline.

528 GOODY TWO (PAIR OF) SHOES ■ Buy two identical-model pair of walking/exercise sneakers at the same time—ideally, at a two-for-one sale at the end of the season. Alternate wearing them. That way you will get more wear out of each pair because they won't be in constant use; they'll have a day to rest in between wearings.

529 INVOLVE YOUR EMPLOYER I: GET A WORKPLACE EXERCISE ROOM ■ Get together with your fellow employees to persuade your employer to turn unused or underused space into an exercise room. The cost to your employer can be as little as $5,000 tax-deductible business-expense dollars for a few exercise bicycles, a treadmill, a complete set of weights, and a large mirror. The benefits of this wellness initiative? Healthier employees, fewer sick days, and possibly even lowered health-insurance premiums.

530

INVOLVE YOUR EMPLOYER II: PAYING FOR YOUR GYM MEMBERSHIP ■ Many employers offer discounts or partial reimbursement for memberships in fitness clubs. Some employers will reimburse you $50–$100 for every six-month period in which you visit the health club sixty times (two or three times a week). You'll be getting paid to keep fit!

531

BRIGHTEN UP YOUR TREADMILL SPACE ■ Most people who stop using their treadmills ditch them because they're boring. But as treadmills can be your key to fitness during the winter, it will pay you to make your treadmill environment more cheerful.

Try some of these to brighten up your treadmill space and encourage its use: a brightly painted room or a poster on the wall, a vase with (artificial) flowers, plug-in scents, or a bowl of potpourri.

532

EASY WALKING LOWERS YOUR BLOOD PRESSURE ■ As people with diabetes are disproportionately susceptible to cardiovascular disease and stroke, discovering that an easy walking program lowers blood pressure enough to make an impact is a godsend.

According to a recent Japanese study, people with high blood pressure who walked as little as 75 minutes a week (three 25-minute walks) lowered their systolic (top number) blood pressure by about 12 points and their diastolic (bottom number) blood pressure by about 8 points in only two months—enough to lower their risk of heart disease.

533

DO THE ONE-MILE WORKOUT WITHOUT LEAVING HOME ■ Bad weather? After dark? No problem. Put on some fast rock 'n' roll and do this snappy routine:

March in place	2 minutes
Side steps, alternating starting foot	3

March in place	1
Knee lifts (march in place with knees raised)	3
March in place	1
Kicking out alternately, the higher the better	3
March in place	2
	15 minutes
Distance	1 mile

534 **OLDER DIABETICS NEED *REGULAR* EXERCISE** ■ Older people with diabetes need to exercise more frequently than younger ones. Mayo Clinic researchers discovered that exercise's effect of increasing the body's sensitivity to insulin may not last very long in older adults. In fact, after four or five days of not exercising, the ability of aerobic exercise to increase insulin sensitivity was still noticeable *only* in people younger than forty. Researchers conclude that you'll need to exercise at least every other day to maintain an ongoing insulin benefit if you are older.

535 **EXERCISE COMBATS METABOLIC SYNDROME** ■ "Metabolic syndrome" is defined as a cluster of common symptoms that dramatically increases the risk of diabetes and cardiovascular disease. Diagnosis of metabolic syndrome requires at least three of these five identifying factors:

▶ Abdominal obesity (a waist measuring over 40 inches for men, 35 inches for women
▶ Elevated triglycerides (150 mg./dl. or higher)
▶ Low "good" HDL cholesterol (less than 40 mg./dl. in men, 50 mg./dl. in women
▶ High blood pressure (equal to or over 130 for systolic—top number—pressure, OR equal to or over 85 for diastolic—bottom number—pressure)
▶ Moderately elevated fasting blood glucose (110 mg./dl.—125 mg./dl., considered the threshold for diabetes

Participants in the large U.S.-Canadian research study rode stationary bicycles for five months. At the end of the trial, one-third of them originally diagnosed with metabolic syndrome no longer had the problem because they had reduced their waistlines, lowered their blood pressure, and improved their lab results. All of these positive changes indicate that exercise can eliminate metabolic syndrome in many people, thus reducing their risk of diabetes and heart disease.

536 COMBINE WALKING WITH HAND WEIGHTS ■ You'll get much more of a workout if you add hand weights to your walking program. Walking at 4 miles per hour with five-pound hand weights is equivalent to *running* at 5 miles per hour. Find weights that feel comfortable in both hands by carrying them around the store for ten minutes before you buy them. (But skip the weights if you have carpal tunnel syndrome or shoulder problems.)

537 WALK BACKWARD, TOO ■ Walking backward gives your hamstring and gluteus maximus muscles the workout that working forward doesn't. So alternate one-minute intervals of walking backward with one minute of walking forward. Find a smooth, safe area, like a building hallway or track, if possible.

538 HALF YOUR WALK, TWICE A DAY ■ Exercising twice a day increases your metabolism and the calories you burn throughout the day. Do half your usual walk in the morning and half after dinner—or maybe five or ten minutes more during one or both sessions.

539 MOVE IT ON UP ■ You may need to increase the iron you are pumping. Light weights will build muscle endurance, but heavier weights will whittle your shape and build solid muscle. Increase the weights slowly and decrease your repetitions. A change from five-pound dumbbells to ten-pounders may be all you need.

540 TAKE SHORTER RESTS BETWEEN SETS ■ Experts recommend taking only fifteen seconds to recover when you are lifting weights for strength straining. That short interval gives you a little rest, but still keeps your heart rate up to burn more calories. (You'll lose that cardiovascular effect if you rest for even one or two minutes.)

541 SHADOWBOX ■ Shadowboxing while you walk works your upper body and improves your posture. Use these moves for one minute at a time, or go freestyle:

Punch out straight in front of you at shoulder height. Next, punch out across your body, again at shoulder height. Then punch overhead. You can do all these punches with one fist and then change sides, or alternate between punches. Improvise!

542 TAKE A HIKE ■ A walking vacation can combine days of serious exertion and cardiovascular benefits with exciting new experiences and the opportunity to make new friends.

Personal story: I went on a week's hike through the Welsh countryside as part of an organized walking tour covering about 60 miles. Because of the hard daily workout, not only was I able to skip one insulin injection a day, but I also lost five pounds despite eating very well.

543 DO LONGER WALKS ON WEEKENDS ■ Try to schedule at least a two-hour walk on pleasant weekends. Most cities and towns have beautiful parks or interesting historic districts. Many even have walking tours—check your weekend newspaper.

For even more fun, turn this into a social event with friends or family, culminating in brunch or dinner.

544 MOVE LATERALLY AS WELL AS FORWARD ■ To increase your workout and involve your inner and outer thigh muscles, add sideways motion to your walk. After a few minutes of walking, turn to the side, take twenty-five sideways steps wider than your shoulder width, turn, and do twenty-five more. Repeat as often as you like, alternating sides.

545 **MAKE YOUR LEGS WORK HARDER** ■ Add lunges to your walk. Step forward on your right foot, keeping your knee over your heel. With your weight evenly distributed between both legs, lower your right thigh until it's parallel with the ground. Push off your left foot to bring your feet together, and then lunge forward with your left foot. Alternate for twelve lunges on each leg, building up to twenty. Repeat this pattern every three to five minutes during your walk.

546 **PICK UP THE PACE** ■ If you can, maintain your walking distance, but increase your speed. If you are presently walking a twenty-minute mile, try for eighteen minutes, then fifteen. Experts suggest increasing your speed twice a week to achieve maximum results.

547 **JUMP FOR JOY—AND BONE DENSITY** ■ As we get older, losing bone density is a problem, and osteoporosis is often the result—for men as well as for women.

Strengthen and protect your bones—and have fun!—by jumping on a trampoline five to ten minutes at a time at least two or three times a week.

548 **RAINY-DAY ROCKABILLY RIOT** ■ It's raining or snowing, and who wants to take a walk in that, or drive to the mall to walk? OK, don't. Let The Killer (or one of his friends) exercise you today. Draw the drapes and put on *any* music by Jerry Lee Lewis; there'll be a whole lot of shakin' going on. Carl Perkins, Chuck Berry, or any of their contemporaries can also get you up and moving. Johnny B. Good!

549

TURN ON A TV PROGRAM THAT TURNS YOU OFF ■ Everyone has a TV show they love to hate—either the political opinions are far from yours, or the sitcom dialogue is moronic, or the ugly contestant can't sing. Let that show inspire you to exertion. Whatever show or film gets your dander up, turn it on and turn it up.

Now give it the talking-to it deserves. Pace, flail your arms, talk back to the set, whatever loud activity gets you going. The dumb pundit won't have learned anything, but you'll feel better, physically and philosophically.

550

BARGAIN WITH THAT FAST FOOD WITH YOUR FEET ■ The quickest path to an insatiable craving is that feeling of denial, so disarm that mechanism *now*. Tell yourself you *can* have whichever fast food is calling your name so loudly—you just need to trade for it. Look through your exchange list and "make room" for what you're craving, but first circle the restaurant twice before you go in. Those few paces accomplish three goals: You'll have exercised a bit; your craving may have eased or even passed during your walk; and, at the very least, you can congratulate yourself for your sense and maturity—before you go ahead and indulge!

6

Dealing with Depression and Stress

551 **LEARN TO LIVE WITH MURPHY'S LAW** ■ Diabetics have a *triple*-barreled right to be angry and depressed. Diabetes is a chronic disease that can last more than fifty years. It requires constant attention and complex treatment, and can have some ugly consequences.

That's the first barrel. The second barrel is the depression that can accompany progress from one stage of life to another. Depression hits extra hard when you're an anxious teenager, a worried parent, or a middle-aged person coming to grips with aging.

The third barrel is Murphy's Law: If anything can possibly go wrong, it surely will.

You can eat exactly the same meal two days in a row. One day it will raise your blood glucose 20 points, one day 100 points. Even endocrinologists don't always know why, and we diabetics get understandably frustrated that the specialists can't explain it to us.

That said, recognize the difference between short-term sadness that has a cause you can pinpoint, and longer-term true depression. After all, as American poet Delmore Schwartz pointed out, even paranoids have real enemies.

Still, if your blues last more than a week or two, call your doctor.

552

GREAT POETRY FOR STRENGTH ■ Find poetry about overcoming the vicissitudes of disease or aging that move you. Some of my favorites:

"Invictus" by William Ernest Henley
"Sailing to Byzantium" by W. B. Yeats
"Do Not Go Gentle into That Good Night" by Dylan Thomas
"Rabbi Ben Ezra" by Robert Browning

553

THE CANINE CONNECTION ■ I've often wondered how many dogs are named "Prozac." Dogs are a marvelous antidepressant for many reasons:

- Your dog loves you unconditionally and shows it often.
- Your dog will make sure that you get out at least twice a day. This will give you fresh air, mild to vigorous exercise, and the opportunity to chat and socialize with other dog owners.
- Your dog lets you be playful and silly, which will lift your spirits.

554

OTHER PETS HELP, TOO ■ Although they may not provide the outdoor benefits, cats and other mammalian pets will cuddle and love you. You can play with them and be silly.

Fish are beautiful, and watching them is a great destresser. Birds are marvelous and some species are extremely intelligent and can be trained to talk. (However, your African gray parrot may outlive you.)

555

FIND AN OLDER, HAPPY ROLE MODEL ■ My ninety-five-year-old aunt Rose is a perfect example. Although she is ill and housebound, she draws and paints, puns, and writes doggerel poetry. Her attitude? "If I wake up in the morning, it's going to be a good day."

556 TAKE A CUE FROM JIMMY DURANTE ■ Legendary nightclub entertainer, actor, and songwriter Jimmy Durante (1893–1980) was a master of the malapropism. The song he used to open his act can inspire all of us:

"You got to start off each day with a song
Even when things go wrong . . ."

Make it your mantra!

557 BUY A SASSY T-SHIRT AND WEAR IT OFTEN ■ One of my favorites has seven silhouettes depicting the rise of man from the apes, starting with what looks like a chimpanzee walking on its knuckles. While the center figure is striding along upright, the last figure is badly hunched over a computer, the caption: "Something, somewhere went terribly wrong."

Other smile provokers: T-shirts titled FEDERAL WITNESS PROTECTION PROGRAM in large capital letters, or anything with the Simpsons or Peanuts characters.

558 CHILD'S PLAY I: BLOW BUBBLES I ■ Think of how much fun you had blowing bubbles when you were a kid. Just the memory should make you smile.

Go to a toy or party store and buy bubble liquid and a wand, or a tube of plastic bubble goo. See what a huge bubble you can make!

If there is no toy or party store nearby and you get the urge, put some dishwashing liquid in a bowl, dip a pastry whisk in it, then blow at the whisk or shake or wave it to make a stream of bubbles.

559 CHILD'S PLAY II: BLOW BUBBLES II ■ The bubble gum of childhood now comes in a sugar-free version. You can order it from many sources on the Internet. Chew and pop that bubble gum and enjoy being a kid again!

560 **HAVE FUN WITH YOUR ENEMIES** ■ Put a picture of your most-hated politician, boss, or ex-love on a dartboard and throw darts at it.

561 **GET YOUR DAILY LAUGHS** ■ Find political cartoons on the Internet. A good site is cagle.slate.msn.com/political cartoons, which offers sixty political cartoons every day, including contributions from eight Pulitzer Prize winners. That's sixty chances to laugh every single day! E-mail the funniest ones to your friends.

562 **GARDEN . . .** ■ Gardening lets you connect with the natural world and create and nurture beauty. You don't need a large plot of land to grow flowers or herbs; even window boxes have enough space. Or grow indoor plants like African violets or cactuses and succulents, or start a sweet potato vine in a jar of water.

Many neighborhoods have community gardens. They are wonderful places to improve your gardening skills and to make new friends.

563 **OR VISIT ONE . . .** ■ Nearly every large city boasts at least one magnificent botanical garden. Turn your visit into a minivacation; arrive early and stay late. Take a picnic lunch and a blanket, a camera and a notebook, a sketchbook and charcoal or pastels. Stroll along the paths and let your mind drift into neutral. Enjoy all the beauty!

Or visit a friend's garden. Offer to help weed or rake to ensure your welcome.

564 **OR BE AN ARMCHAIR GARDENER** ■ If the preceding tips are inconvenient, be an armchair gardener. Borrow gardening books from the library. Get seed and plant catalogs. Research specific gardening issues on the Internet.

Are you more ambitious? More creative? Plan your dream garden on graph paper, or on your computer, or sketch it. One day you may achieve it!

565 **VOLUNTEER AT AN ANIMAL SHELTER** ■ Any kind of volunteering is good for your soul. When you volunteer at an animal shelter, you usually feed and water the animals, play with them and pet them, getting them used to being touched by loving hands.

Walking shelter dogs is a pleasant chore. You get to socialize with several dogs at every visit and also get a lot of exercise you don't have to think about.

566 **TRAIN YOUR DOG TO BE A THERAPY PET** ■ Calm, friendly, well-behaved dogs between the ages of one and ten make ideal therapy pets. After evaluation and a training session, you and your dog will be visiting nursing homes, hospitals, and rehabilitation centers, improving the quality of life for institutionalized patients. Dogs provide excellent rehab opportunities. Patients who refuse physical therapy will gladly throw a ball for your dog, or walk him. Autistic or withdrawn patients are happy to talk to him. And your volunteering will make you glow!

567 **GET ENOUGH SLEEP** ■ Sleep deprivation is a major cause of depression. Most adults need eight to nine hours of sleep a night; a few need as little as seven or as much as ten. Without naps, very few people are alert and happy on only five or six hours of sleep.

Catching up on your sleep on weekends doesn't work very well. You really need to get a good night's sleep every night. Try going to bed a half hour earlier for a week, then an hour earlier. See if you're not more cheerful!

568

DON'T LET S.A.D. SADDEN YOU ■ S.A.D. (Seasonal Affective Depression) is the medical term for winter blues, the depression that occurs because the days are shorter and often bleak and gloomy.

Take advantage of every sunny day to get out and walk for at least a half hour. But if the sun is strong, use a sunscreen or sunblock and wear sunglasses.

If you live in an area with few sunny winter days, you might want to purchase lightbulbs that are designed to mimic sunlight.

569

START BUILDING YOUR CASTLE ■ Borrow your children's Lego blocks or Lincoln Logs, or buy them used in thrift shops, flea markets, or yard sales.

Get down on the floor and have fun!

570

YOU ARE NOT A NUMBER ■ Do you remember *The Prisoner,* the groundbreaking fantasy series of the late 1960s, in which Patrick McGoohan (No. 6) frequently cries out, "I am not a number, I am a free man!"

You, too, are not a number. You are much more than your blood-glucose number or your glycohemoglobin A1C number, which may be high and which may depress you. You, too, are a free person, and you are free to improve your numbers.

Don't let the "numbers game" get you down. You are a whole person, a unique individual.

571

PLAY A KAZOO ■ The kazoo is an inexpensive musical instrument that can be learned very quickly and takes no talent whatsoever to play well. Maybe that's why it's been around since 1884, according to Webster's dictionary. All you have to do to make music is hum through the tube.

If you get the urge and there's no toy store near you, just put a tissue paper over a comb and start humming.

572 **APPLY A COCKAMAMIE** ■ Even the name makes me smile. It's a corruption of the word "decalcomania," which we New York kids had probably never heard and couldn't have pronounced. In other words, a temporary tattoo.

Applying them now can bring us back to childhood, or can be used for a devil-may-care or erotic gesture. Put them where the world can see them, or just a special someone. They'll last for about five days, but you can wash them off earlier if you get tired of them. My favorites are Harley-Davidson logos—all the swashbuckling and bravado, none of the pain.

573 **TAKE A MINICRUISE** ■ There's something wonderfully soothing about being on the water—even for just an hour or two. Most cities on lakes, rivers, or oceans offer a variety of inexpensive water trips, sometimes combined with dinner, music, a historical tour, or even whale watching. Even an off-hour commuter ferry can be fun.

When you return, you'll probably feel refreshed and better able to focus.

574 **READ BIOGRAPHIES FOR INSPIRATION** ■ People who have accomplished great things or made momentous discoveries—often in the face of poverty or disability— can inspire us to overcome our own problems that we thought were insurmountable.

Read the lives of the great geniuses—Ludwig van Beethoven or Thomas Alva Edison—whose creative output was astonishing despite their deafness. Of Winston Churchill, who battled his "black dogs" of depression as well as World War II's Axis Powers. Of Mother Teresa, who fought poverty and disease as well as the orthodox Roman Catholic establishment.

Although not a biography in the strictest sense, the letters of Vincent Van Gogh—mostly to his brother Theo—are extremely revealing and inspirational.

575 **COLLECT A LIBRARY OF FUNNIEST FILMS** ■ You might want to start at the American Film Institute's Web site, which features the 100 Funniest, or list your own favorites and build your collection. Some personal favorites: *The Producers,* Marx Brothers' outrageous classics *Duck Soup* and *A Night at the Opera,* the screwball comedy *Bringing Up Baby,* W. C. Fields's last starring film, *Never Give a Sucker an Even Break,* featuring the world's most hysterical car chase, and the Christopher Guest mockumentary, *Best in Show.*

Relax for a couple of hours, pop one of these classics in your VCR, and convulse with laughter.

576 **GO BACK TO SCHOOL** ■ Increase your knowledge or learn a new skill at your local community college or Y. Hundreds of courses are available every semester. Learn a foreign language, develop your creative skills, or study a subject you always wanted to when you were younger.

577 **TEA CAN GET YOU THROUGH** ■ The British standby, "a nice hot cup of tea," has seen millions through all kinds of adversity. It may be the calming liquid, but it's also probably the ritual. Late in the afternoon, you stop everything and break for tea. When you return to work or your daily chores, everything seems clearer, more manageable.

578 **VARY YOUR DAILY ROUTINE** ■ Do you always walk or drive along the same route? Do your laundry on the same day of the week? Maybe that's what's getting you down.

Change your daily routine a little. Take a different route to or from work. Save your chores for a different day of the week. Better yet, list how many aren't really necessary—and don't do them until next week or next month.

579 **DON'T BE YOUR OWN WORST ENEMY** ■ Ditch unreasonable expectations for yourself. They are a major cause of chronic depression, which makes your diabetes worse and more difficult to control.

Cut yourself some slack. Be as forgiving with yourself as you are with your best friends. Make two lists: "Five Things I Like About Myself" and "Five Things I'm Proud Of." Keep them in your wallet and look at them frequently.

580 **SMILE AT YOUR NEIGHBORS** ■ The physical act of smiling is a powerful antidepressant.

Smile at neighbor children and at people walking their dogs. Engage them in conversation. You will feel less isolated, and you may learn new things.

581 **BUY YOURSELF FLOWERS** ■ Flowers are an inexpensive indulgence. In Manhattan, a little judicious shopping will get you two dozen roses for only $10.

Two dozen roses is a lavish gift from you to you in appreciation of your existence. Take the time to arrange them gloriously in one or more vases. Steal one rose for your night table, another for your bathroom. Enjoy all this natural beauty!

582 **LEARN FROM THE SERENITY PRAYER** ■ The great American liberal theologian Reinhold Niebuhr's Serenity Prayer has been a mantra for millions of people who try to live by these simple, profound words: "God grant me the Serenity to accept the things I cannot change, the Courage to change the things I can, and the Wisdom to know the difference."

Focus on the Serenity and Courage, and your mood will lift.

583 **FIND BEAUTY WITH A KALEIDOSCOPE** ■ A kaleidoscope isn't just a kid's toy. You can use it to facilitate
meditation and find your "quiet place." Rotate the collar, and the
brightly colored bits of glass turn into the mesmerizing rose windows
of Notre Dame Cathedral in Paris.

A teleidoscope works the same way, but uses just a lens and mirrors
which reflect and multiply whatever you point it at, much the way a
fly's eye works, so you will see real objects broken into myriad planes,
making fascinating patterns.

584 **ROSEMARY CAN REV YOU UP** ■ Hamlet's Ophelia
may have shortchanged rosemary; she praised it only
for "remembrance." The herb's aroma fights fatigue by triggering the
release of norinephrine, a brain chemical that lifts energy levels. It also
increases beta brainwaves, associated with alertness.

585 **BRIGHT COLORS LIFT YOUR SPIRITS** ■ Depression
feeds on black clothing. Think of all the negative figures of speech associated with "black," versus "being in the pink."

But don't dump your basic black. Perk up your wardrobe, ladies,
with bright-colored scarves and jewelry; men, with bright or cartoon-
motif ties.

You'll feel better when you look into the mirror, and other people
will respond to you more positively.

586 **WEAR FRAGRANCE** ■ Fragrance has the power to
banish the blues. When you wear cologne or after-
shave, you automatically feel more attractive to yourself and to the rest
of the world.

You can intensify this feeling by wearing an old favorite that you
wore years ago. Here's why it works: Olfactory (scent)-evoked nostal-
gia, as scientists call the term, is so strong because there is a direct

connection between the olfactory bulb at the top of your nose and your hypothalamus, the brain's memory center. No other sense has such a direct connection to your brain. When you wear a favorite old fragrance, you can remember all the happy, intense emotions you experienced when you wore it in the past.

587 THE LURE OF LEMONS ■ Did you ever wonder why furniture polish and other household products contain lemon oil? Lemon smells good, and it's also energizing. Experts say that lemons' scent molecules contain turpine, a biochemical that increases alertness by stimulating the trigeminal nerve, the principal sensory nerve of your face.

Enjoy fresh lemon peel in potpourri. Mix equal parts of lemon peel with chopped lemongrass, dried lemon verbena leaves, or rosemary. When your potpourri loses its fragrance, pour it into your bath to release the last of the scent.

588 HEADS UP! ■ Actors know how to create character through posture and physical movement. They express confidence and alertness with an upright head and forceful physical actions. They express depression with a hangdog posture and hesitant movement.

Learn from actors. When you keep your head up and move confidently, your movements will make you feel less depressed.

589 BREAK THE BAD POSTURE = PAIN + DEPRESSION CHAIN ■ Poor posture leads to migraines and back pain, and pain is a major cause of depression. Spending hours at a time hunched over a computer keyboard can cause what orthopedists call "postural syndrome" or "postural derangement," which can trigger neck, shoulder, and back pain, and the resultant depression. It's hard to be happy when you're hurting.

Breaking this chain is not difficult, but it requires developing and practicing new habits. Start by taking thirty-second breaks from the computer to stand up, stretch, take a few deep breaths, and stand very straight, like the military "attention" posture.

More structured exercise, like yoga or Pilates, will help you achieve pain-free good posture, too.

590 **FIND A MANTRA** ∎ Mantras—words or phrases repeated as invocations or incantations—have destressed millions of people over the centuries and helped them focus. One or more of these may work for you:

"Om"
"Peace"
"I believe."

My favorite: the Biblical "And it came to pass," because of its eternal wisdom and perspective. The Bible never says, "And it came to stay."

591 **READ A SACRED WORK** ∎ Holy books have consoled us and strengthened our faith for thousands of years through their enduring wisdom.

Read the Old or New Testament, the Koran, the Upanishads, or the Bhagavad Gita. Or, if you do not feel traditionally religious, you may feel more comfortable—and comforted—with the Book of Psalms or the *Meditations* of Marcus Aurelius.

592 **ATTEND RELIGIOUS SERVICES** ∎ These, too, can banish depression and stress and lift your spirits.

Being part of a community of worship also strengthens your feeling that you are not alone in this world.

593 COUNT YOUR BLESSINGS ■ When you focus on your blessings, you realize that your cup is half-full, not half-empty.

Be thankful for family and friends, for your job or profession, for your home, for all the things that you enjoy. Write them down—you'll be surprised at how many you can list.

594 FOLLOW YOUR BLISS ■ Mythologist and folklorist Joseph Campbell, subject of the Bill Moyers PBS special *The Power of Myth,* coined the phrase "Follow your bliss" to describe the burning need that individuals and societies have to identify what they are passionate about.

Following *your* bliss leaves little room for depression and stress. Passion and excitement drive them out and create an environment for happiness.

595 WIDEN YOUR CIRCLE OF FRIENDS ■ One of the consequences of modern life is an extremely mobile population. Nowhere is it more visible—or more psychologically damaging—than in how long our friendships last. Personal story: Within the last three months of 2003, my two best friends moved from my Manhattan neighborhood: one to Long Island, the other to Orlando. As a result, I'll probably see them once or twice a year instead of once or twice a week.

Widening your circle of friends protects you from suddenly losing your best friends. Here's another example of safety in numbers!

596 LIGHT CANDLES ■ Most of the world's great faiths use candles in their religious rituals. They symbolize light in the darkness, hope in a world of uncertainty.

You, too, can benefit from the symbolism of candles. You can use them to focus when you are praying or meditating. Or they can banish the blues in winter. They also create a festive atmosphere, and that, too, can generate happiness.

597 JOIN A SUPPORT GROUP ■ Support groups give you *many* brains solving problems and sharing experiences. And their discussions often spark creative new ideas. They are definitely worth trying. And if your first support group isn't helpful or has some obnoxious participants, try other groups.

598 USE MESSAGE BOARDS ■ Message boards offer all the advantages of support groups, plus two more big ones: anonymity and the flexibility of visiting and contributing only when it is convenient for you.

599 DO THREE GOOD DEEDS A DAY ■ This should be a desirable goal, not an inflexible rule. Good deeds take you out of yourself and can help you forget your diabetes for a while. Your good deed can be a little thing, like holding a door or an elevator for someone with a lot of packages, or phoning a friend or neighbor just to touch base. Or it can be something major, like visiting a shut-in or a hospitalized friend, or helping a neighbor who has a toddler *and* an infant.

Whatever good deed you do, *you* will feel better as a result.

600 FIND YOUR QUIET PLACE ■ Your quiet place can remove your stress. It can be real—a favorite armchair or the bathtub, or mental—Tahiti, or even imaginary—Middle Earth.

What counts is that you can send your body or your mind to that magical center to drift and relax. You will return refreshed and destressed.

Note: If your imagination could use some inspiration, try guided-imagery tapes.

601 VOLUNTEER ■ Every community needs volunteers, and volunteering is a more structured way of doing three good deeds a day.

Most cities and towns can use hundreds of volunteers, so your choices can be wide. Check with your mayor's office or your city's Web site for options.

602 TREAT EVERY DAY AS A GIFT ■ Since our national disaster of September 11, 2001, most of us are mindful that life is uncertain. Make the most of each day. Regard it as a golden opportunity to do something special, to be someone special.

603 FOCUS ON THE PRESENT AND THE FUTURE ■ No one can change the past. You can learn from it but you can't change it, and it's self-destructive to obsess over it and to play the "If only I had/If only I hadn't" game. And self-destructive behavior creates stress and leads to depression.

Instead, focus on the present and the future. What can you do today, this week, this year to improve your health and your life?

604 MEDITATION BEFORE MEDICATION ■ Western medicine is pill oriented. Antidepressants are a billion-dollar market. But many people with diabetes don't like taking another batch of pills on top of the diabetes, cholesterol, and stroke-prevention medications they are already taking.

Try meditation first. Find your quiet place and let your mind wander. Experiment and see which technique works for you. If you feel less depressed after a couple of weeks, you may not need antidepressant medication at all.

605 MEDICATION DOES NOT MEAN FAILURE ■ Because every person has a unique brain chemistry, antidepressant medication may turn out to be the best solution. If pills work better for you than meditation or other therapies, do *not* regard it as a personal failure—that's just the way your brain is wired.

Make your goal "Whatever works for me."

606 WATSU MAY WORK FOR YOU ■ What is Watsu? A trademarked abbreviation of "water shiatsu," a therapy that combines therapeutic massage with water's healing properties.

Developed at a California hot-springs retreat in the 1980s, Watsu is now practiced by many massage therapists. Clients start in a pool of 98-degree water, the same as your body temperature. The warm water and gravity-free environment induce deep relaxation and help your spine and tense muscles let go.

Massage is the second part of the session. Many clients who experience Watsu find that it drives out feelings of tension, rage, depression, and stress.

607 DRESS FOR SUCCESS ■ Any form of discomfort can induce or add to already-existing stress. Avoid tight, overly restrictive clothing or clothing that is too loose or too baggy. Clothing that fits comfortably and is neither too warm nor too lightweight will make you feel better, look better, and be more relaxed. If the environment of your workplace differs markedly from the outdoors, dress in layers.

608 IT'S STRESS, BUSTER ■ Your job is often a cause of stress. Sometimes taking a break and walking around the block will do wonders to alleviate your stress. Any mild exercise will often do the trick, but Type A people have to remember that it's not a contest, and end up creating more stress by overdoing it.

609 USE A TOUCHSTONE TO BEAT WORKPLACE STRESS ■ A touchstone, in this context, is an object that you pass by frequently during your workday. Your personal touchstone might be a plant, a photograph, or even the water cooler. After you choose your touchstone, put your hand on it whenever you pass it and keep it there for a couple of seconds. Let it remind you to breathe more deeply, to focus, to take a short break. This technique, called "grounding" or "anchoring," helps to reduce stress.

610 ALWAYS HAVE A "PLAN B" ■ It's a fact of life that few things go according to schedule. Curveballs abound.
If you are not flexible and don't have an alternative plan, you're going to get stressed out. Having and following a "Plan B" will prevent that from happening.

611 SILENT NIGHTS LOWER STRESS ■ Living in a noisy neighborhood can raise your stress level, especially when you sleep. As a survival mechanism, most people's auditory systems are still working when they are asleep, on the alert for sounds that signify danger. A noisy environment increases the production of your stress hormones.

Why is that important? Excessive blood levels of the stress hormone cortisol have been linked to an increased risk of aging and disease, especially insulin resistance and cardiovascular disease.

What can you do about it? The easiest solution is to wear earplugs. If they don't work for you, try a radio station that plays soft music or a machine that plays a continuous tape of a waterfall to drown out the noise.

612 STATINS MAY REDUCE DEPRESSION RISK ■ Statin drugs like Lescol (fluvastatin), Mevacor (lovastatin), Pravachol (pravastatin), and Zocor (simvastatin) are used to lower cholesterol and are being prescribed for people with diabetes even if their cholesterol is low or normal because the drugs can cut the risk of cardiovascular disease and stroke in diabetics by about one-third.

Now it appears that statins may also lower depression risk when they are used continuously for years. After average use of four years, patients on statin therapy had a 30 to 40 percent reduced risk of depression and lower levels of hostility and anxiety. Every additional year of statin therapy lowered these risks even more.

613 NOBODY'S PERFECT—AND THAT MEANS YOU ■ Insisting on being perfect, especially in minor things, is a recipe for major stress and for the depression that results because you're *not* perfect. No one is!

Give yourself permission to put most issues and tasks into the "not really all that important" category. Remember that the best baseball players in history struck out more than 70 percent of the time.

614 FIGHT DEPRESSION I: STAY FIT ■ Physical fitness helps the body to help the mind. Feeling better and having better flexibility, strength, and endurance and more energy will go a long way to make your outlook more positive, more confident, more able to cope with everyday problems and hassles. *Mens sana in corpore sano!* (A healthy mind in a healthy body.)

615 FIGHT DEPRESSION II: STAY ACTIVE ■ Maintaining a routine will alleviate boredom, which feeds depression. Having other things to think about, having things to look forward to every day, will help you avoid aimlessness, which is one of depression's greatest allies.

616 FIGHT DEPRESSION III: STAY FOCUSED ■ The mental aspect of fighting aimlessness is not letting your attitude slide any more than your physical activity does. Live your life each day, and keep your goals in front of you, even if it's only a trip to the local store. Don't talk yourself into procrastination.

If you have problems staying focused, make a "to do" list the night before. Number your chores and check them off as you complete them.

617 FIGHT DEPRESSION IV: STAY COMFORTABLE ■ Physical discomfort magnifies depression. Almost all brainwashing techniques begin with physical discomfort, not outright pain. Make sure your living space is warm enough, that your clothes aren't too restricting, that your shoes are comfortable, that you have enough of the right food to eat. Take care of the physical body, and that will help take care of the mind.

618

CREATE A PLEASURABLE WAKE-UP RITUAL ■ Enjoyable early-morning rituals will destress you and help you face the day.

Do your windows face east? Sleep with your window shades up and let the sun wake you.

Awake to the aroma of freshly brewed coffee by programming your coffeemaker the night before. Almost as good as having a butler, isn't it?

Set your clock radio to your favorite music station—maybe even a little early so that you can hit the snooze alarm and still be on time.

619

UNWIND AFTER WORK ■ When you get home, take a five- or ten-minute break. Kick back, take off your shoes, and put your feet up on the nearest piece of furniture. Take a few deep breaths and let them out slowly.

That short break is all it takes. Now you can face the rest of your day without carrying over any workplace stress.

620

GETTING READY THE NIGHT BEFORE ELIMINATES MORNING STRESS ■ After dinner, listen to the weather forecast, then lay out tomorrow's clothes. Are they clean and pressed? No buttons missing? No open seams? Shoes polished.

Next pack your briefcase or backpack with everything you'll need and get tomorrow's lunch ready if you're brown-bagging it.

Tomorrow morning should go smoothly, with no unwelcome little surprises. And you'll have removed a major source of stress.

621

HIGH BLOOD GLUCOSE RAISES YOUR STRESS LEVEL BY AFFECTING YOUR THINKING ■ You knew that *low* blood glucose (hypoglycemia) clouds your thinking and raises your stress level because your mind just isn't working well. But did you realize that *high* blood sugars alter your thinking almost as much? Even short-term spikes in blood glucose can sap your mental sharpness, verbal ability, and mathematical skills.

Avoid stress by keeping your blood-glucose levels as even as possible.

622 **CONNECT WITH NATURE** ■ Take a few minutes to look—really look—at a flower, a tree, a bird, a squirrel. Notice how the sunlight strikes the buds or shines through the translucent petals or filters through the leaves.

If you are observing a bird or a squirrel, stay very still and they may approach you out of curiosity. (Or lure them with sunflower seeds. Squirrels also love M&Ms.)

In connecting with nature during this brief, quiet interval, you will be letting your stress flow out of your mind and body.

623 **A CATNAP CAN BE YOUR CATNIP** ■ Even the briefest nap can revive you, lower your stress, and lift your spirits. The great Winston Churchill attributed his clear strategic thinking, energy, and boundless optimism during the crises of World War II to his frequent daily catnaps.

Let catnaps work for you, too!

624 **READING DRIVES OUT DEPRESSION** ■ Listen to the words of essayist and philosopher Michel de Montaigne (1533–1592), arguably the greatest mind of the French Renaissance, who sometimes got depressed, too:

"When I am attacked by gloomy thoughts, nothing helps me so much as running to my books. They quickly absorb me and banish the clouds from my mind."

Don't they strike a chord in us more than four centuries later?

625 **MAKE BILL PAYING LESS ONEROUS** ■ Let's face it: No one enjoys paying bills. But using illustrated checks can make the chore less burdensome.

You can choose from more than one hundred designs, including comic-strip characters, animals, flowers and landscapes, and Bible verses. My personal favorite: vintage Harley-Davidson motorcycles.

626 **SWAP HATED CHORES WITH A NEIGHBOR . . .** ■ Chances are you don't hate the same chores equally, so trade off with a neighbor.

One of you cleans both your ovens, the other washes and waxes both your floors. Before Thanksgiving, one of you hand-washes both precious china and crystal collections, the other polishes your silver and your friend's.

Isn't this a less stressful way of handling the chores you hate?

627 **. . . OR HIRE A NEIGHBORHOOD KID TO DO THEM** ■ Most kids need more spending money than their allowances give them, and they are willing to work for it.

Benefit from their energy and strong muscles by hiring them to do the chores you dislike the most.

628 **WALK ON AIR** ■ One of the fastest, easiest, and least expensive treatments for depression and stress may be a pair of gel insoles for your shoes. They make walking easier and put a spring in your step. And when your feet are happy . . .

629 **STAY OUT OF DEBT** ■ Financial problems can worry us day and night, draining our mental and physical energy. That's a prime recipe for depression and stress.

Creating a realistic monthly and yearly budget is a crucial first step.

Include categories for savings and leisure. Careful planning will help you avoid living from paycheck to paycheck.

630

CUDDLE WITH THAT SPECIAL SOMEONE ■ Act like a teenager again and cuddle on the living-room couch. Express your loving feelings! Share your dreams and plans.

631

MASSAGE YOUR NECK AND SCALP ■ Do you feel a tension headache coming on? Defuse that stress by massaging your neck and scalp.

Start at the back of your neck with the fingertips of one or both hands. Move your fingertips in small circles, using as much pressure as you're comfortable with. Then move your fingertips in small circles all over your scalp. This will increase the flow of blood to the area and minimize the likelihood of a full-blown tension headache.

632

PRACTICE RANDOM ACTS OF KINDNESS ■ The gospel "Practice random acts of kindness and senseless acts of beauty" was created by Ann Herbert in 1982 and has since spread around the world.

Many cities celebrate a Random Acts of Kindness Week during the second week of February with special projects and programs.

For suggestions as to what you can do on this special week or every day, log on to the Random Acts of Kindness Foundation Web site: www.actsofkindness.org. You can find dozens of other wonderful ideas at www.helpothers.org.

633

SOLVE PUZZLES ■ Stimulating your brain is a wonderful antidepressant.

Puzzles are ideal because many types are so portable. All you need for them is a pencil or a pen. You can pick them up whenever you have a few minutes, then put them down again. Try crosswords, acrostics, or jumbled words.

When you have more time and space—like a rainy weekend—you may want to try solving chess problems or doing jigsaw puzzles.

634
WORK SMARTER, NOT HARDER ■ Start every task by thinking for a few moments. Is there a better or easier way to do this job? Saving time and effort will make you feel so much better!

635
LIGHTEN YOUR TO-DO LIST ■ Many of us make a to-do list every morning, or the night before if we're extremely organized. Then we check off every item on the list after we do it.

That's very organized—but honestly, now, are all of these tasks absolutely necessary? If you had time to do only five or ten of them, would this particular task still be on your list? Could you eliminate it? Postpone it? Combine it with another task?

Or, if you prefer the words of the visionary business consultant and philosopher Peter F. Drucker, "There is nothing so useless as doing efficiently that which should not be done at all."

Now that you have an expert's permission, do something happy and relaxing with the time you've freed up.

636
GIVE YOURSELF A SPA DAY ■ Don't wait for your love or your kids to give you a gift certificate. And it won't be necessary to empty the piggy bank. This is something you can do for yourself at home for less than $10.

Start with a facial—guys, too. Use a grainy soap like oatmeal and almond and a loofah sponge. Follow up with a masque suited to your skin type. Spread it over your face, avoiding your eyes, and remove it with a warm washcloth. Then apply a moisturizer. You'll look and feel much younger! Just peek in the mirror.

Now take a long soak in the bathtub. Put a cup of oatmeal in a cut-off pantyhose leg. Save the orange peel from breakfast, cut it into small pieces to release the fragrant oils, put the pieces into the pantyhose leg, knot it, and toss it into the tub. Fill the tub with water as hot as you can stand it and get in with a magazine or paperback. Stay in for at least twenty minutes and just relax.

After you get out of the tub, put on sweats or comfortable old clothes. Give yourself a manicure and pedicure, or just slather cream on your hands and feet and put on cotton gloves and socks for an hour. Put your feet up.

Spend the rest of the day just relaxing.

637 JOIN A BOOK CLUB ■ Participate in a book club with a small group of people who read the sort of books you enjoy, whether it be literature, modern fiction, fantasy and science fiction, travel essays, poetry, et al. Reading a book to discuss it is a very different experience from reading a book on your own; take notes while you read so that you can discuss the book intelligently.

Some people like to join book clubs where a kind of book they *don't* usually read is discussed, so as to open up new genres for their enjoyment.

Most book clubs read a book a week or every two weeks. If you can't form a club from among your friends, most independent bookstores as well as the large chains offer congenial groups.

638 MUSIC LIVE OR ONLINE ■ Let live music lift your spirits. Go and see local musical groups perform in cafés, coffee shops, and bookstores—almost always for free. Splurge on tickets for the opera or Philharmonic.

If you're an online type, take advantage of the wonderful songs on iTunes. Even if you can't afford to buy a lot, sometimes listening to 30 seconds of that oldie you remember from years ago is enough to give a lift to your day.

639 KEEP A JOURNAL ■ Write regularly in a journal. It can help center you and organize thought processes that may seem chaotic at the time.

640

DELIGHT IN ONLINE COMICS ■ Subscribe to an online comics update. It will send amusing and dramatic comic strips to your in-box every day. A good one is http://www.unitedmedia.com/comics. It's nice to have something to laugh at every day!

641

THE TAO OF DANCING . . . ■ Take dance lessons. Even if you don't care much about dancing, the lessons can be wonderful for putting you more in touch with your own body, making you feel more in tune with yourself and more graceful at a time when you might feel angry at your body for letting you down.

642

. . . AND OF YOGA ■ Yoga classes can often provide the same benefits as dance classes, with the added advantage that many will teach you how to meditate and center yourself. Choose a class at a yoga center, *not* one given by a gym, unless you want to use the class merely for exercise. Choose a form of yoga that will concentrate on its mental and spiritual benefits, such as kriya, siddha, or sahaja yoga.

If you are new to yoga, kriya yoga utilizes a methodology of self-reliance, self-discipline, self-inquiry, and meditation, which induces direct perception into the nature of consciousness and the individual's thinking patterns.

Siddha yoga focuses on spiritual awakening, self-realization, and balance. Sahaja yoga is a method of meditation based on self-awakening and the spontaneous union with the self.

643

TAKE A LITTLE RISK ■ No, not skydiving without a parachute or riding your bike without a helmet, but doing something that's a little bit of a stretch for you.

Maybe it's just buying a lottery ticket once in a while, or taking a three- or five-mile hike if you're not sure you can go the distance.

What counts is opening yourself to new experiences.

644 **LOOK UP AN OLD FRIEND** ■ You lost touch years ago; you may not even remember exactly when or why. Perhaps one of you moved or changed jobs.

Make today the day to reconnect. Grab your Rolodex or address book and pick up that phone!

645 **START A KAFFEEKLATSCH** ■ Get together with some friends, neighbors, or coworkers once a week for coffee. No agendas, just socialize and enjoy your time together.

646 **BOYS'/GIRLS' NIGHT OUT** ■ It doesn't have to be at night, either. Just a group of guys or gals having fun together.

647 **GROOM YOUR PET** ■ Spend five or ten minutes a day to comb or brush your pet. Use long, slow strokes. Look into his eyes and have a one-sided conversation.

Hasn't *your* blood pressure dropped? Don't *you* feel better, too?

648 **RENT A THREE-HANDKERCHIEF MOVIE** ■ Sometimes you need a good cry when you feel depressed or stressed. The best way to release your feelings is to rent the kind of film that legendary directors called a "three-handkerchief movie."

Here are some personal recommendations to start you off:

The Elephant Man
Equus
I'll Cry Tomorrow
It's a Wonderful Life
On Golden Pond
Stella Dallas
Torch Song

649

THE JOY OF FINGERPAINTING ■ You don't have to be able to draw to take advantage of the joyful experience of fingerpainting.

This is your opportunity to be spontaneous—even messy. To connect with your Inner Child. Doesn't it feel wonderful?

Save your best efforts. Post them on the refrigerator or even frame and hang them.

Added bonus: You'll smile as you walk by them.

650

BE CAMERA READY ■ Spend a morning or afternoon with your camera in a park or historic district of your town. For this little adventure, buy a disposable camera for around $5 at your local drugstore.

Pretend that you are a photography student on assignment to take the most unusual pictures, and don't go home until you finish the roll.

Won't you be surprised when you see the developed pictures!

651

ONE HUNDRED STROKES ■ Ladies, did your grandmother train you to brush your hair one hundred strokes every night?

This old-fashioned beauty ritual requires bending at the waist and dropping your head. This move alone will relax your neck muscles and increase the flow of blood to your head and neck.

Then, with a natural-bristle hairbrush, brush your hair from the roots to the ends, following each brushstroke with a similar stroke from the palm of your opposite hand. This motion counts as one stroke.

Concentrating on the brushing and the counting will free your mind. And not only will this ritual destress you, but your hair will become much glossier and your complexion will glow more.

652

BREATHE EASY ■ A great deal of our daily stress is both the cause and the result of shallow breathing.

We are stressed, so we don't breathe deeply. And because we are not taking in enough oxygen, our bodies are not functioning at their best, and we become stressed.

Break this vicious circle. At least once every hour, breathe as deeply as you can. Feel your lungs filling up, all the way from the bottom to the top. Take at least five breaths this way every hour.

At the end of a week, ask yourself whether you've felt less stressed. The answer will likely be yes.

653 THROUGH A CHILD'S EYES ■ Seeing the world through a child's eyes can reawaken your sense of wonder. To a young child, even the most mundane events and experiences are novel. If you do not have small children or grandchildren of your own, borrow a neighbor's child for an hour or two and see what both of you discover!

654 PLAY TOURIST IN YOUR OWN TOWN ■ Many New Yorkers have never been to the top of the Empire State Building or ridden the Staten Island ferry. Many San Franciscans have never toured Muir Woods or the wine country.

Don't take interesting things for granted or skip visiting them just because they're in your own backyard. Ask your convention and visitors' bureau for a list of the top sights, maps, and travel directions. There may even be some discounts and freebies in the package they send you!

655 CLEAR CLUTTER QUICKLY ■ Innocent little pieces of paper can gang up on you and drive you nuts—especially when they pile up everywhere and you are trying to find one specific item—like a bill, a prescription, someone's business card, a child's report card.

Trying to locate that one piece of paper wastes your time, and that creates major stress. You also feel as stupid as all get-out, which is very depressing.

Here are a few ways to eliminate clutter:

▶ Sort your mail at the wastebasket. Toss anything that isn't important. If you live in a building with a mailroom, don't even carry junk mail into your home. Just throw it away immediately.

▶ Put all your bills into a brightly colored folder so that you can find them quickly when you have to pay them. Put anything that requires your immediate attention into the same or another brightly colored folder.

▶ Put almost everything else into *one single box* and deal with it every week. *Never let it overflow;* that's how you got into trouble in the first place.

▶ Use refrigerator magnets for appointment slips, prescriptions, and laundry tickets.

656 **SIMPLIFY YOUR LIFE** ■ This concept is broader and more profound than merely lightening your to-do list (Tip No. 635).

Think about what is really important to your life, versus what you can get along without. The excesses of Hollywood celebrities and Wall Street tycoons assault us every day through the media, But even without the collection of 100 vintage cars or 1,000 designer gowns, some of us are pack rats on a smaller, more modest scale, with 3 or 4 cars and 50 pairs of shoes.

Are all your possessions really necessary, or is it time to give away or sell some of them? Remember: What you don't have, you don't have to store, clean, or insure.

657 **USE THE FIVE-DAY WEATHER FORECAST** ■ Paying attention to the five-day forecast can simplify your planning. If you have a home-based business and live in an area where the weather varies greatly, take advantage of pleasant days to run errands and meet with clients and friends. Use nasty weather for phoning prospects and clients and working on detailed projects that need long periods of concentration.

658

GO BAREFOOT WHERE IT'S SAFE ■ Few mood-lifters beat going barefoot. Therapists would probably say that it's a psychic return to a happy, carefree childhood. Walking barefoot in your home is safest, and wiggling your toes into plush carpets and fluffy rugs is pure, sensuous delight.

If your toes and feet are normally sensitive, it may also be safe to walk barefoot on your lawn or on a pristine beach. Keep on wiggling those toes and feel like a happy kid again! (And examine your toes and feet carefully afterward.)

659

GO ON A SCAVENGER HUNT ■ You'll need two people or two evenly matched teams for this creative game.

First, have each person or team list ten unusual items on a piece of paper. Next, exchange lists and agree on a time for the hunt to end and a meeting place.

Now off you go on your hunt! No swiping allowed—if you need someone's property, get permission to borrow it and make sure you return it without damage.

The winning person or team is the one who collects the most items or, if there is a tie, the most unusual choices.

660

HAVE AN UPSIDE-DOWN DAY ■ Just for fun, make a weekend day an upside-down day. Have your dinner for breakfast—you may need to adjust your medication—and your breakfast for dinner. If you usually wear casual clothes, dress up, and vice versa.

How many other things can you do to shake up your routine a little bit?

661

ENJOY THE SEASONS ■ First snowstorm of the season? Build a snowman or have a snowball fight with your kids or your love. Or just throw the snowballs at a tree or a wall to check out your pitching arm.

Spring? Visit some of the big-city flower shows or botanical gardens. Pick up some ideas for houseplants or your garden.

Summer? Get into a hammock or a rocking chair with some sugarless lemonade or diet soda. Ree-lax!

Fall? Go to the best or nearest place to see the leaves change color. A weekend trip with a night at a country inn would be lovely, but a drive through your neighborhood can also fill you with beauty.

662 TRY AN UNUSUAL WEEKEND ACTIVITY ■ As they used to say in *Monty Python's Flying Circus,* "And now for something completely different. . . ."

Shake up your weekend routine by trying something unusual for you. Do you like to visit museums or see movies? Go to a ball game instead or organize a potluck dinner with some friends. Plan your next vacation—real or imagined. Wander through an antiques show or hit the yard sales. Check the weekend edition of your newspaper for more ideas.

663 VISIT A COMEDY CLUB ■ The Comedy Channel offers lots of laughs, but visiting a comedy club is much better. There is much more spontaneity, outrageousness, and topicality—and far less censorship. And there's always the chance that you'll see a major new talent at the beginning of his or her career.

664 REALITY CHECK I: TEN THINGS YOU LIKE ABOUT YOURSELF ■ When we're depressed—and people with diabetes frequently are—we focus on the negatives, not the positives. We see the glass as half-empty, not half-full.

So here's a reality check to put things in perspective. Sit down and make a list of ten things that you like about yourself. They can focus on your appearance, your achievements, or anything else. But you *must* come up with ten. (If you need inspiration, ask your family and friends.)

665 **REALITY CHECK II: TEN THINGS YOU WANT TO CHANGE ■** Now it's time to focus on the future. Think of what you'd like to change. Maybe it's as simple as a hairstyle or color, or as complex as a career change.

Again, sit down and list the ten things you want to change. Remember: You can always make changes in your life.

666 **REALITY CHECK III: IF YOU HAD ONLY ONE YEAR TO LIVE ■** And now here's the most intimate and challenging exercise. What would you do if you had only one year to live? How would your priorities change? What would become the most important things to do? What would you dump?

Of course, you have much more time. But separating the truly important from the trivial is necessary to get joy out of life.

Remember the old Latin motto: *Carpe diem* (Seize the day).

667 **MAKE A SEXY PHONE CALL ■** OK, you've been serious and soul-searching long enough. Now it's time to inject some fun into your day. Make a sexy phone call to the person you love most. It could go like this:

"This is an official obscene phone call. Know what I'm gonna do to you tonight? First I'm gonna chew off all your buttons, kissing you in between each one. And then I'm gonna kiss you up, down, and sideways. And then . . ." *You* fill in the blanks if you're not both already giggling.

668 **CREATE A CARTOON WALL ■** Collect your favorite cartoons, frame them if you're feeling craft-y, and hang them on a wall. Use magnets to put them on the refrigerator or inside your front door.

I like putting cartoons into Lucite shadow-box frames because it's so easy to slide out old favorites and slide in new ones to create a constantly changing gallery of fun.

669

CONSIDER A CAREER CHANGE ■ Very often unhappiness with your job is at the root of your depression or stress. Here are some things you can do about it:

If your own job gives you grief but the company and benefits are good, check with your company's bulletin boards or make a friend in the Human Resources Department and see if there are other, better jobs you might qualify for. Network with friends at other companies; maybe they're hiring. Start reading the weekend help-wanted ads or look on the Internet. Polish up your résumé.

Or, given the trends in outsourcing, maybe this is the time to go into business for yourself! (I did thirty-two years ago.)

670

MUSIC'S "VALIUM EFFECT" ■ Classical music has been shown to work as well as Valium. In one study, listening to thirty minutes of classical music had the same tranquilizing effect as 10 mg. of Valium. Drift and soothe yourself with Pachelbel's *Canon,* Ravel's *Bolero,* or chamber music by Bach, Haydn, or Mozart.

671

MULTITASKING CAN STRESS YOU ■ Do one thing at a time before moving on to the next job. Eliminating distractions and focusing on the task at hand will help you complete it more quickly and accurately. And focusing on one thing at a time will make you feel less stressed.

672

CARVE OUT AT LEAST ONE HOUR A DAY FOR YOURSELF ■ Create a sanctuary at home. Teach your kids to keep out when the door is closed, except in emergencies. (If they can close their door, why can't you?)

Don't answer the phone—that's what answering machines are for. This is *your* time, for just unwinding.

673 TEMPER, TEMPER ■ Here's a powerful reason to lower your stress level. Men who are generally hostile or frequently angry may have as much as a 30 percent greater risk of developing such irregular heart rhythms as atrial fibrillation, a risk factor for stroke, according to the Framingham Offspring Survey. Hostility did not appear to increase heart disease in women, but researchers believe that stress can also impact men's and women's general and cardiovascular health by influencing them to practice unhealthy habits.

674 MINDFULNESS MEDITATION REDUCES STRESS ■ Like other forms of meditation, mindfulness meditation is an exercise in centering. In mindfulness meditation, you become deeply aware of the present moment, a practice that reduces stress and may boost immune-system function, according to a study reported in the July-August 2003 issue of *Psychosomatic Medicine*.

To practice mindfulness meditation, sit quietly for ten to twenty minutes, clearing all thoughts from your mind. Close your eyes and breathe deeply and evenly.

675 MAYBE YOUR STRESS IS JUST EYESTRAIN ■ Your stress may be caused by simple eyestrain. If your stress disappears when you close your eyes or gaze out of the window for thirty seconds, eyestrain may be the culprit.

When was the last time you had your vision and your eyeglasses checked? (People with diabetes should see an ophthalmologist every six months and an optometrist at least once a year.) Your eyeglass frames may need a little tightening or adjustment so that your eyes are looking through exactly the right area of the lenses.

Quick fix: Soak cotton balls in witch hazel, and place the compresses on your eyelids for five to ten minutes. Even better, keep the bottle of witch hazel in your refrigerator between uses.

676 **COLOR YOUR HAIR** ■ Gray hair can be depressing. It makes us realize that we are getting older and, visually, gray hair can wash the color out of your face.

Temporary hair colors that last through three or four shampoos are available for men as well as for women. Try one and, if you like the results and start receiving compliments from your friends and family, try a permanent hair color. Life is too short to have gray hair!

677 **COLOR YOUR ENVIRONMENT** ■ Colors awake strong emotional responses. Savvy people use them as antidepressants. You can make the boring blandness of a white or beige room or apartment disappear without even painting it by creating happier moods with inexpensive accessories.

Decades of research in the psychology of color shows that colors have the power to evoke moods:

Blue—the most soothing, peaceful, and nurturing color.
(Remember the blue of the Madonna's robe.)
Green—serene, suggestive of gardens, forests, the natural world.
Red—warmth, excitement, drama.
Yellow—sunlight and optimism.

Add splashes of color to your rooms easily and quickly by hanging stained-glass suncatchers in your windows, collecting cheerful coffee mugs, choosing new towels, throws, and decorative pillows, and even—for maximum variety at minimum cost—stocking up on coordinating paper plates and napkins.

Perk up your workspace with a funny cursor and a beautiful screen saver.

678 **UPDATE KO-KO'S LIST** ■ First a little background: In Gilbert and Sullivan's *Mikado,* Ko-Ko, the Lord High Executioner, rattles off a delightful patter song, cataloging all the types

of people who irritate him, concluding each verse with "They'll none of 'em be missed."

The original song dates from the 1850s, but its concept is even more timely today, and invites us to destress ourselves by updating Ko-Ko's list with our own pet peeves.

For inspiration, here is master parodist Keith Peterson's witty update:

"There's the movie palace patron with the intermittent cough;
The pest who owns a PDA and never turns it off;
The diner who is less than prompt at reaching for the check;
The broker who promotes a stock because it ends in '-tech';
And women in department stores who fill your lungs with mist—
I rather doubt the mist is likely to be missed!"

Now you try it—you'll feel a lot better!

679 WATER WORKS I: PLUG IT IN ■ Fountains have a hypnotic quality that soothes us and lifts our spirits. Fountains have such a positive effect on us because the circulating water raises the levels of negative ions (the air's electrically charged particles) that make our spirits soar. You can find a small fountain with a compact circulating pump for your home or garden for less than $75.

680 WATER WORKS II: CRYSTAL CLEAR ■ Water in glass containers concentrates light and energy, according to the Hindu design philosophy *vastu*. For optimal effect, arrange clear vases filled with water in powerful groups of three to represent the life-force triad: wind, water, and fire.

681 HANDLE CURVEBALLS WITH STYLE ■ Life is full of potholes and curveballs. The key to your overcoming them is being flexible, rather than rigid. We all had grandmothers who dealt successfully with unexpected guests or tiny food budgets by adding more water and spices to the "always magically full" soup pot.

Or friends who perfected the art of the five-minute straighten-up by piling everything behind the shower curtain.

You can always find solutions if you innovate!

682 DEPRESSION IS UNDERDIAGNOSED IN MEN ■

Millions of men in the United States suffer from undiagnosed depression. Although 6 million men in the United States are estimated to have a depressive disorder, many health professionals believe that many—if not most—may never be treated for it. One large study found that 75 percent of people seeking professional help for serious depression were women, but 75 percent of people in the same group who committed suicide were men. The study concluded: "Women seek help—men die."

Men, this may be a wake-up call to do some serious soul-searching. If you've been feeling unhappy or anxious for more than two weeks, tell your doctor that you think you may be depressed, and ask for help.

683 PRACTICE COGNITIVE RESTRUCTURING ■ We often

tend to "awfulize" situations. Little things get magnified all out of proportion. Your train is late two days in a row, and you automatically jump to thoughts that your boss is ready to fire you.

When negative thoughts like this become an automatic response, they can lead to hypertension, depression, and other physical and emotional problems.

Cognitive restructuring (CR) is a mental technique that lessens negative thinking. It teaches you to think in context instead of "awfulizing." To practice CR, begin by saying "Stop!" to yourself. This breaks the cycle of negativity. Then take two or three deep breaths and let them out slowly.

Next, give yourself a reality check: Are you seeing the situation in the worst possible light? Are there other ways to look at it? A better, more probable perspective?

Finally, take positive action: Is there an intelligent way to deal with this problem? Then do it!

684 STOP THE "FAT AND UGLIES" ■ Geneen Roth, author of *Feeding the Hungry Heart* and *Wł. ᷄ ᷄ood Is Love,* an expert in emotional eating, has come up with "the fat and uglies," a concept that many people with diabetes are familiar with, and which increases their feelings of worthlessness and desperation, making them want to pig out beyond belief.

According to Roth, we don't know what triggers the syndrome— only that we feel so unloved that we retreat to food, the only thing that *does* love us.

The best way to disarm the fat and uglies is to have an internal monologue with your fault-finding self. Agree with it, and you'll destroy its power. Say to yourself, "Yeah? So what?" when it starts ranting that you're fat and ugly. When you realize that, you can avoid emotional eating, move on, and feel like your own, good, valuable self again.

685 CHEAP PAMPERING I: MAKEUP MAKEOVER ■ Ladies, this one's free and lots of fun. Visit a department store—especially during seasonal promotions—and get a makeup makeover. Let one of the makeup artists apply new products and colors. Usually, you're not obligated to buy anything, but you may be tempted to treat yourself to a new lipstick to coordinate with the season's hot colors.

686 CHEAP PAMPERING II: MINIMASSAGE ■ You don't need to spend an hour or $60 to $80. Many massage therapists provide ten-minute minimassages for $10, which may be all you need to relax your neck and shoulders and make you feel marvelous. You can find massage therapists who offer these quick treats in many malls and parks, or through the American Massage Therapy Association, www.amtamassage.org.

687 CHEAP PAMPERING III: TRANSFORM YOUR BATHROOM ■ A bathroom that appeals to your senses can feel incredibly pampering, and it can be done inexpensively. Here are some ideas to get you started:

- Spray-paint a handful of pebbles gold, so that they resemble gold nuggets. Arrange them in a clear glass dish on your sink counter.
- Or take some pretty shells or some colored pebbles for an aquarium and place them in the dish.
- Buy several cakes of scented soap. Some—like lavender or oatmeal and almond—are unisex.
- Pick up a few loofahs and some deep-sea sponges in different sizes and textures.
- A little more expensive, but definitely worth it: a new showerhead with a variety of pulse and spray options so that you can customize every shower you take.

688 CHEAP PAMPERING IV: DRESS UP YOUR BEDROOM ■ You can make your bedroom feel very special, too, and make its inhabitants feel very pampered. Try these ideas:

Put a vase with fresh, silk, or synthetic flowers on your dresser. Or—for a touch of drama—use four or five peacock feathers.

Place sachets in your dresser drawers, or line them and your closet shelves with scented paper. Here, too, lavender is an excellent unisex choice.

For a little splurge, pile a collection of decorative pillows on your bed. You can usually find them on sale at home-decor shops.

689 HAVE YOU FORGOTTEN WHAT *YOU* WANT? ■ Curiously, it is both a cause and an effect of stress that you may have forgotten what you like—or would like—to do. Call it "the caregiver syndrome": We are so busy taking care of other people that we forget about ourselves.

It's time for you to focus on yourself. It may have been so long since you've done so that you need some help. List-making time:

▶ Is there anything you used to enjoy doing and would like to do again? Anything new you'd like to try? List three films you'd like to see, three books you'd like to read.
▶ Jot down the names of friends you'd like to see more often.
▶ Write down three places where you'd like to vacation.

690 **TEACH YOUR PARTNER OR KIDS TO DO HOUSEWORK** ■ Stop being everyone's maid. It's time your family pitched in—they live here, too, and they dirty your home up, too.

Many men do dishes and laundry. Teach yours to vacuum, too. Kids can set and clear the dining-room table, load up the dishwasher, and even prepare dinner if they're old enough. Everyone over the age of seven should clean the bathtub after using it.

You can probably come up with a chore list more appropriate to your own family and home. This should start you thinking.

691 **HEAD FOR THE PARK** ■ A nearby park or playground offers a great escape, ideal for making your stress disappear.

Get on the swings. Climb on the monkey bars. Have fun on the seesaw.

If you're fortunate enough to have a park with a merry-go-round, take a couple of spins and relive your youth.

692 **WHISTLE AWAY STRESS** ■ Whistling, humming, or singing can melt away stress. Here's why this happy habit works: The sound-frequency patterns you create by making music trigger positive changes in your alpha brain waves, which relax you.

693 **BEAT STRESS—GET ORGANIZED I: STASH YOUR KITCHEN TOOLS** ■ Putting your most frequently used kitchen utensils in a widemouthed jar or crock keeps them handy. Tools like tongs, spatulas, a soup ladle, a grater, baster, melon bailer, wooden spoons are easily findable in a crock, much less so if you have to rummage for them in a kitchen drawer. In fact, you can probably identify them just from their handles.

694 **BEAT STRESS—GET ORGANIZED II: ALPHABETICAL ORDER SAVES TIME** ■ This isn't a sign of obsessive-compulsive behavior. Alphabetizing your spices and herbs saves you search time every time you cook.

695 **BEAT STRESS—GET ORGANIZED III: DOUBLE YOUR KITCHEN CABINET SPACE** ■ Using two-tiered turntables not only doubles your cabinet space, it also makes everything on them equally accessible. That's a big timesaver.

696 **BEAT STRESS—GET ORGANIZED IV: TOTE YOUR SUPPLIES EASILY** ■ Store your cleaning supplies in a caddy under the sink and tote them easily from room to room. You'll free up precious overhead shelf space.

697 **BEAT STRESS—GET ORGANIZED V: SIMPLIFY YOUR CLEANING ROUTINE** ■ Jot down your cleaning routine on index cards and post them on your fridge with a magnet. Try new cleaning products or methods that are supposed to save you energy and time once, then decide if they're worth adopting permanently.

698 **BEAT STRESS—GET ORGANIZED VI: KEEP BACKUPS** ■ Have at least one extra set of house and car keys—two sets are even better. Have alternate ways to get to work, to get the kids to school, several alternate babysitters.

699

BEAT STRESS—GET ORGANIZED VII: KEEP ADDRESS-BOOK PAGES BY FUNCTION AS WELL AS NAME ■ Add extra pages to the front of your address book and list similar people there so you can find them quickly. For example, one page might list all your doctors, the dentist, and the pharmacy, with all their addresses and phone numbers.

On another page, all the parents in your younger child's playgroup. A third page might list all your older child's teachers and half a dozen classmates. On a fourth page, your boss and some coworkers. On a fifth page, your mortgage holder, insurance agent, electrician, plumber, painter, handyman, and mechanic.

Isn't that a faster, easier way to find people?

700

BEAT STRESS—GET ORGANIZED VIII: DUPLICATE IMPORTANT DOCUMENTS ■ Birth certificates, marriage certificates, car titles, real estate deeds, passports, and insurance policies should be protected in a safe-deposit box. Keep copies of these documents in a large plastic bag or envelope with a watertight closure. In a disaster, just grab it and go.

701

BEAT STRESS—GET ORGANIZED IX: NIGHTSTAND NECESSITIES ■ Keep these items on your nightstand within easy reach: telephone, flashlight, pens or pencils, and a pad. You may also want to add an index card with the emergency phone numbers of people who are very important to you.

702

BEAT STRESS—GET ORGANIZED X: WHEN YOU TURN THE CLOCKS, DO THESE ■ Changing your clocks back and forth to daylight saving time and standard time is a good time to do these important little chores: change the batteries in your smoke detector, and throw out expired medicine and sunscreen.

703 BEAT STRESS—GET ORGANIZED XI: CLEAR YOUR DESK ■ If you don't need it today, put in your desk drawer. Keep it off your desk—you'll concentrate better.

However, if those papers and files overflow that desk drawer, it's a wake-up call that you need to do some major organizing.

704 BANISH TOXIC PEOPLE FROM YOUR LIFE ■ Toxic people depress us. They make us unhappy. Their negative energy poisons everyone and everything around them. If someone or something is 95 percent wonderful, toxic people will focus on and criticize the other 5 percent.

There's a simple solution: Recognize that only a miracle (or therapy?) will change these toxic people, so banish them from your life. You'll be so much happier!

705 LEARN TO SAY NO ■ Some people are such givers that they become stressed. They are overscheduled and overburdened.

If you are one of these wonderful people, learn to say no. It's an act of self-affirmation and empowerment.

Listen up if you're not used to saying no:

Learn to say "I'm sorry, but I can't." Period. No explanation. If someone presses you to explain, just repeat, "I'm sorry, but I can't."

Eventually your questioner will back off.

End of your stress.

706 HAVE NO REGRETS ■ Life is really too short to have regrets. As the eternally beautiful Sophia Loren is reported to have said, "I have no regrets. Regret only makes wrinkles."

707 PLAY THE INVENTOR ■ Let your imagination run wild. What kind of product or gizmo is missing from your life set? Can you make it from scratch or cobble it together from things you already have? Think about it, sketch it, and maybe even make it!

708 MAKE YOUR APPEARANCE A POSITIVE ■ When you feel better, you think and look better, which makes you feel better, and so on. If you feel terrible—for emotional, physical, spiritual, or any other "reasons—clean up and dress up. Putting yourself into a downward spiral at any point will have a domino effect. Especially if you're irritated or disgusted with yourself over food or exercise promises not kept, pulling your visible self into shape gives you more strength and motivation to begin the next step of getting where you (or your doctors!) want you to be.

709 PUT YOUR BELIEF TO WORK FOR YOU ■ Countless studies have shown that optimism can extend lifespans. Optimists tend to outlive pessimists, and people with religious beliefs tend to last longer than atheists. A positive outlook can make enormous differences, and using that inner strength can make managing blood-glucose levels much easier. If you ever gave up a beloved food for Lent, or stopped eating bread during Passover, then you know how much easier small self-denials can be when they're made for a Greater Cause.

710 SUPPORT NETWORKS MAKE ALL THE DIFFERENCE ■ How many people love you? How many do you love? How many do you tell, and hug, and have contact with every week? Research studies show that people with strong networks of intimate social contacts are healthier, happier, and stronger, longer. If social situations are difficult for you, consider joining a club for one of your interests. Being in a room full of other bridge or chess players, or slot-car enthusiasts, or quilters, or pastry chefs, gives you many automatic conversation openings. And those contacts can boost your immune system as much as they lift your spirits.

711 **WHEN YOU CAN'T DO ANYTHING ELSE, RELAX** ■ A positive attitude is more than optimism and a smile— it's sometimes the only thing you can do to make a situation better. Studies show that emotional resilience is one of the most important qualities you can bring to your wellness and your quality of life. So after you've done all you can, if there's nothing else you can do, relax and see where the flow takes you. Stressing yourself to no benefit will only make your situation worse.

712 **LIMIT THE DAMAGE BY ADJUSTING YOUR LIFESTYLE** ■ You are in control—not of everything, not of every detail. But you are in control of the *limits* of your diabetes, and that's a mantra worth repeating. What you eat, how much you exercise, whether or not you smoke or drink to excess—these things accelerate or delay complications of diabetes. In the moments when you feel restricted or resentful, remember: In large part, as much as you are willing to accept the responsibility, you are in control.

713 **PROMISE TO BE SMART AND HEALTHY** ■ Tell the truth: Don't you keep promises to other people better than you keep promises to yourself? Most people do, so use it. Promise someone special that you'll develop new health habits. For many people, keeping that promise is easier because it has another person attached.

714 **GET TOUCHED BY AN ANGEL** ■ The lovely overseeing angel in the former TV series, *Touched by an Angel,* wants to help other people with diabetes. Actress and ordained minister Della Reese was diagnosed with type 2 diabetes several years ago, and has written "Be Stronger Than Diabetes," an inspirational pamphlet to help others manage their diabetes. You can get a free copy by logging on to www.delladiabetes.com.

Undeniably, the best antidepressant and destresser is a loving relationship. To keep your love growing and glowing, try these easy ways to get romantic. I hope they inspire you to create your own rituals!

715 **GET ROMANTIC I: STARGAZE** ■ On a clear summer evening, spread out a blanket and sit under the stars. Look up at the heavens and share your dreams for the future.

716 **GET ROMANTIC II: BREAK A SWEAT TOGETHER** ■ Sweating is sexy. The aroma of your love can be a real turn-on. Go hiking or running together, or do some heavy housecleaning together.

717 **GET ROMANTIC III: CELEBRATE SILLY ANNIVERSARIES NOW** ■ You may or may not reach your golden anniversary—so celebrate it now—just the two of you—with a special trip, or something you've always wanted to do.

Or celebrate the anniversary of the day you met, your first date, or any occasion that's meaningful to you.

718 **GET ROMANTIC IV: READ LOVE POETRY TO EACH OTHER** ■ Great poetry is *very* romantic, and there are thousands of beautiful, sensual poems to read from.

My personal favorites for a romantic evening: Chilean poet Pablo Neruda's *100 Love Sonnets (Cien sonetos de amor),* in a bilingual edition, Shakespeare's sonnets (154 to sample!), and poetry by e. e. cummings, Edna St. Vincent Millay, Robert Graves, Edward FitzGerald's many translations of *The Rubaiyat of Omar Khayyám,* and the poems of Catullus.

Take turns reading to each other and enjoy the voice of your beloved!

719 **GET ROMANTIC V: SAY IT'S YOUR HONEYMOON** ■ If you're going on vacation, you can often get VIP treatment from hotels, tours, and cruise lines if you tell them it's your honeymoon. Champagne, gift baskets, a free spa visit have all been reported by happy couples.

720

GET ROMANTIC VI: START A COLLECTION TOGETHER ■ It doesn't have to be expensive or *Antiques Roadshow* or *Incurable Collector* quality. What counts is that you're doing something pleasurable together and learning together.

Start by making the rounds of yard sales and thrift shops to see if anything appeals to you—especially objects that you'd like to collect in quantity. There are lots of interesting, attractive items you can buy in the $10–$50 range that may possess long-term investment potential.

721

GET ROMANTIC VII: DO AN APHRODISIAC DINNER ■ I won't discuss the nutritional value of my suggestions here, although they definitely exist. What's important is their delicious decadence and their deserved centuries-old reputations as aphrodisiacs. Also, as you don't want to expend hours in the kitchen, you can get this entire meal together in less than a half hour.

brut (dry) champagne—domestic is fine.
caviar—salmon roe is tasty and inexpensive.
lobster or crabmeat salad—make this the day before with canned
    crabmeat, if you're on a budget.
fresh strawberries—even if they're out of season. Dipping them
    in bittersweet chocolate before you feed them to each other
    will make them even more decadent!

722

GET ROMANTIC VIII: SPEND A DAY IN BED WITH YOUR LOVE ■ The best for last! Lock the door and turn off the phone. 'Nuff said!

7

Tips from Children with Diabetes and Their Parents

723 **GET SOME SUPPORT** ■ Nobody will understand your situation and frustrations like another parent with a diabetic child—and you may not need to invent any wheels somebody else has already covered. Log on to http://www.childrenwith diabetes.com for an online community for kids, families, and adults with diabetes. News of breakthroughs, upcoming conferences, nutrition, summer camps, basics, and warning signs—this is a fine Web site to start with or return to.

724 **FINANCIAL HELP IS AVAILABLE IN EMERGENCIES** ■ Families struggling to pay for diabetes supplies can apply for short-term assistance from Supplies for Children with Diabetes. Children with type 1 diabetes who are in emergency situations—like the loss of health insurance, loss of a parent's job, or a local disaster—can get supplies for up to three months, one month at a time. This program is part of the Children with Diabetes Foundation. For more information, log on to www.cwdfoundation.org/Supplies.htm.

725 **YOUR CHILD'S DIABETES REQUIRES COOPERATION FROM CAREGIVERS** ■ If your child is in day care or school, make sure that your child's teacher knows you need their help with reinforcing healthy eating habits away from home. Schools with cafeterias publish their daily menus ahead of time; offer healthy snacks to share with the class on days when it's your child's turn to bring in treats. And send him off armed with a healthy lunch and snack on days when the school's foods aren't appropriate for his diet.

726 **BECAUSE YOU'RE THE PARENT—THAT'S WHY** ■ Frustrating and inconvenient as it can be sometimes, you're a grown-up, and it's important to help your child manage diabetes successfully. Teaching your child how to eat properly now will set patterns that will help manage his diabetes for the rest of his life.

The healthy eating plan you adopt for your diabetic child can be good for your entire family to follow. Your commitment to your child's present and future well-being must be full-blown and full-time. Even more than telling him what's right and counting his exchanges and helping to monitor his blood-glucose levels, you need to display behavior worthy of modeling. Eat your six-plus servings of fresh fruits and vegetables every day. Skip the gravy on your entree, so he sees that it's tasty without the "goo." And if you must have a candy bar, indulge when your child is in school or somewhere else that you're not. He'll learn much more from what he sees you *do* than from what he hears you *say*.

727 **WATER: YOU GOTTA LOVE IT** ■ Teach your child to drink water as the beverage of choice. Good hydration helps the body control blood-glucose levels, and water also helps limit carbohydrates from other beverages. Drinking 8 ounces of orange juice is the carbohydrate equivalent of eating two oranges; choosing 8 ounces of water instead will do your child twice as much good.

728 **WHAT A FRIEND WE HAVE IN FIBER** ■ There are many reasons why increasing your child's fiber intake will benefit his body. Your grandma told you about roughage; enough said there! But in addition to moving waste through the intestines more quickly, high-fiber foods are more satisfying because they are so filling. They are digested more slowly, and they keep blood-glucose levels more consistent for longer.

Give your child more fiber without his even noticing. Try substituting high-fiber foods like whole-grain bread or cereal, beans, and popcorn for white breads, sugary cereals, and potato chips.

729 **MAKE TV A DIRTY WORD** ■ Studies show that the more time kids spend watching television, the more likely they are to be overweight—and eat poorly. These are the key causes of the epidemic of *type 2 diabetes* in children and adolescents.

Make TV a treat, blocking out time only for certain shows or special occasions. Give each child his own color highlighter and mark TV listings for the one or two shows the child really wants to see. In addition to limiting sedentary viewing time, there's an added bonus: Your child learns to set priorities and limits by ranking chosen favorites over "whatever's on at 7:00."

730 **BAN EATING IN FRONT OF THE TV** ■ Make this a family rule, and keep it: no eating anyplace except the kitchen or dining-room table. Snacks in front of the tube are doubly deadly: Not only are you and your kids zoned out and sedentary, you're also taking in calories that are almost certainly carbs and fats. (Admit it: *Nobody* eats celery sticks in front of the boob tube.) And unless you have a dog to police the area for you, those Cheetos in the sofa cushions are the perfect bug-bait!

731 **SNEAK SOME VEGETABLES PAST YOUR KIDS** ■ Even if they "hate vegetables," you can disguise them and slip them into other dishes, and they won't even know they're eating healthier.

Add cut-up extra vegetables to chili or stir-fry dishes. Grate root vegetables like carrots and rutabagas and add them to stews. (Don't sneer until you've tried it—you really won't taste them!)

Your skin will start glowing, too!

732 FRUIT FIRST ■ "As soon as diabetic toddlers develop teeth, switch them from (diluted) juice to chunks of fresh fruit. They will enjoy manipulating this new finger food, and fresh fruit has more nutrients and fiber than juice, and won't make their blood glucose rise as rapidly because it is digested more slowly.

Save the fruit juice for their hypoglycemic episodes.

733 YOUR CHILD'S MEDICATION WILL CHANGE ■ As kids grow, they gain weight. Their diet changes, and so may their activity level.

Diabetic kids are no different. Any one of these changes will affect their insulin and other drug needs.

Phone your child's pediatrician or endocrinologist if your child is starting a growth spurt, beginning school, or if you simply find that your child's formerly predictable blood-glucose readings are yo-yo-ing.

734 LET *ALL* THE TEACHERS KNOW YOUR CHILD'S NEEDS ■ Diabetes requires a great deal of monitoring and self-care. Diabetic schoolchildren often depend on teachers and staff to provide the encouragement and support they need to take care of themselves. Be sure your child's teachers—*all* of them, not just homeroom—know that he needs extra bathroom breaks, and specific times to check blood-glucose levels or have a snack.

Don't let an overworked teacher or snippy administrator tell you they can't take on any additional obligations—schools have a legal responsibility to accommodate the special needs of children with diabetes.

735 DIABETES AT SCHOOL CAN MEAN MORE THAN SNACKS AND MONITORING ■ Diabetic children may need special understanding: Their concentration can wander, and occasional behavior difficulties can arise out of rapid changes in blood-glucose levels. Make sure that your child's teachers or day-care providers are educated about your child's potential emotional as well as physical needs—your child's misbehavior may not come from the same motivations as other children's, and needs to be addressed differently because the remedy and resolution come from different needs. Make sure your child receives fair treatment from his teachers and school.

736 GET INFORMATION OR HELP FOR YOUR CHILD'S SCHOOL ■ "Discrimination" sounds like an odd term for diabetic schoolchildren, but many of today's overcrowded and over-burdened school systems don't look forward to "special-needs students." You may need to educate yourself as to your child's legal rights, and enlighten the school personnel about their responsibilities toward your child. Children with diabetes have to be medically safe at school and in day care, while having the same access to educational opportunities as other children. The American Diabetes Association and the Juvenile Diabetes Association provide educational materials for both parents and school personnel to understand how to meet the medical and academic needs of students with diabetes. (See Tips 777–779 for details.)

737 YESTERDAY'S LEVELS ARE HISTORY—CHECK AGAIN AND AGAIN ■ Children's blood-glucose levels need to be checked often because their levels of play and food intake change so frequently. Until you establish a regular schedule, you'll know best how often your individual child needs to be checked by watching her mood and behavior, energy output at play (active versus sedentary), or even by noticing the smell of her breath or urine.

Teenagers' body chemistry is in almost-constant flux, so expect that puberty may cause even more variation in blood-glucose levels, calling for more frequent testing.

738 PLANNING A "FAMILY SWEET" TWICE A WEEK TAKES THE STING OUT ■ Few things spark cravings more strongly than the feelings of restriction or denial. Help your child moderate her consumption of sweets by planning special desserts once or twice a week, and making a family event out of sharing them. (You can decide whether a low-carb or no-sugar-added dessert is all right for other nights of the week.) By also encouraging half-size portions, your child can feel included in a collective celebration and still indulge a bit. And knowing that she's "saving up" for when the entire family can share the occasion can help with self-control at other times during the week.

739 WHAT YOUR CHILD *DOESN'T* EAT ALSO MATTERS ■ Remember to give yourself points for what your child *didn't* eat today. While what he *did* consume is what shows up on the glucose meter, every sweet or fatty food that *wasn't* eaten would have caused more trouble in his arteries or capillaries in another decade. Controlling your child's food intake can be an overwhelming job— especially if the child isn't cooperating much yet—and parents may need to acknowledge themselves for how good a job they do, especially on a day when they feel the job could have been done better.

740 YOUR OWN RESCUE STRATEGY ■ Keeping a level head is as important—and sometimes even more important—than keeping level blood-sugar numbers. Some parents report that the enormity of monitoring a child's blood glucose and medications 24-7 hits them hard periodically.

Just as you have insulin or orange juice ready in case your child has a crisis, be sure you have your own "emergency fix" at hand in case you feel the blues coming on. A parents' support group, someone who can give you half a day off, even a half-hour massage can make an immediate difference in your equilibrium. Keeping yourself on an even keel is the best thing you can do for your child. Just like the airline attendants' instructions, put your own oxygen mask on first so you can be in a position to assist your child.

741 EVEN LITTLE CHANGES CAN MAKE ENORMOUS DIFFERENCES ■ Small changes in growing children can reap enormous long-term health benefits. In preadolescent children, every inch they have yet to grow will be accompanied by pounds they have yet to gain. If a child can gain a little less weight as he approaches his final height, that growth will actually be realized as a *weight loss*—achieved more easily than weight loss will ever be again, as an adult.

742 PUBERTY: A TOP TIME FOR TYPE 2 ■ A steady relationship with a good pediatrician or doctor is vital during your child's growing up. Puberty in prediabetic children can bring on more body changes than the ones you'd expect. The body is more insulin-resistant during puberty, and the growth spurts and weight gain during that time strain the body to produce more insulin than it can manufacture. Type 2—insulin-resistant—diabetes can be the result, which gives your child that much more to cope with during an already-stressful part of life.

743 DIET, EXERCISE, AND INSULIN ARE THE ONLY TOOLS FOR TYPE 2 KIDS ■ Children who develop type 2—insulin-resistant—diabetes have three easily accessed tools with which to fit it: diet, exercise, and insulin. Unfortunately, they are the *only* tools: The oral medications adults can use to assist insulin uptake are not approved by the Food & Drug Administration for use in children.

The most recent surveys show that one in four American children is seriously overweight—more than one in three in some ethnic groups like Mexican-Americans and Native Americans. As a result, children are increasingly developing what was once called "adult-onset" diabetes, and may need to take insulin injections for a while, until their blood-glucose levels are stabilized, the FDA is currently studying Glucophage (generic name metformin) for use in children, but it has not yet been approved.

744 **NEW DIRTY WORDS: "ESCALATOR" AND "ELEVATOR"** ■ Trade no-effort conveyances for stairs whenever possible. Escalators and elevators burn no calories and contribute nothing to cardiovascular health. Young children can play counting games, taking stairs two at a time, or one step for each syllable of a song; older children can be "dared" or "raced" up steps. Since five flights is daunting for anyone, promise your child that you'll climb one flight and then take escalators or elevators the rest of the way. Eventually, try alternating climbing one flight and riding one floor until you've reached your destination. Don't forget to praise *any* new effort: The eight or ten steps in a flight of stairs really *is* a big accomplishment for a heavy child.

745 **THE REAL "BARGAIN" IS PAYING FOR ONLY WHAT YOU NEED** ■ The suggestion to "supersize" is everywhere, and twice as many French fries for just 39 cents more sounds like a real bargain—especially to a youngster who's good at math. The problem is that neither you nor your child *need* that many, and there's an extra 300 or more calories in that larger portion. If some inner sense of thrift urges either of you to buy the bigger one because it "costs less," think again. Redefine "bargain" as "getting exactly what I want and need for my money." If paying a little for a lot more still excites you, then supersize your sugar-free drink and ask for a courtesy cup. Share it with your child, and both of you can skip the fries!

746 **YOU ARE WHAT YOU DRINK** ■ Many overweight children are telling the truth when they protest, "But I don't eat that much!" Unfortunately, kids today think nothing of downing 32-ounce "Big Gulp" drinks—the equivalent of four servings. Merchandisers have accustomed us to giant helpings, which now look normal and make 6- and 8-ounce drinks look midget sized. Teens who down two 32-ounce drinks a day have consumed one-half gallon of liquid, and even if it's fruit juice—don't let it be soda pop!—that's still an enormous amount of calories and sugar. If you're determined to fork over money for a drink in a container for your child, try low-fat milk or bottled water.

747 HALF-NUDE BURGERS ■ The hardest part of dietary restrictions for kids can be the sense of not being included—not being able to go to the same places and eat what their friends eat. So if a fast-food place is where the gang is going, diabetic teens can have their hamburgers along with everyone else. Just have them ask for no "special sauce," and jettison half the bun. Using it like a holder, or like peeling a banana, they can tear away the bread as they eat the meat. If any jerky companion questions the practice, just have your child say, "It's soggy, it's too gross to eat." Nobody argues with "gross!"

Better yet, have your kid toss both halves of the bun!

748 THE RISKS OF CHILDHOOD TYPE 2 DIABETES ■ Complications from type 2 diabetes can occur at any time, but it's worth remembering that some complications might not crop up until twenty or thirty years later. When an adult develops type 2 diabetes in his forties, that means troubles in his late sixties and seventies. But when a fifteen-year-old has high blood-glucose levels, high cholesterol, and high triglycerides, that means a thirty-five-year-old will be facing life-or-death problems related to diabetes.

If you can see the sense of saving now for your child's college expenses, then it surely makes sense to take steps now to fend off his possible cardiovascular and stroke problems just ten years after college.

749 IT'S NOT "JUST A COLD" ANYMORE ■ Diabetic children's colds and viruses are different from other children's even if it's the same germ. Over-the-counter medicines affect blood-glucose levels and blood pressure differently in children with diabetes, and parents of diabetics shouldn't try to self-medicate when they're sick. It's not trivial—call your pediatrician, and monitor often.

750 EVERY KIND OF SICK ISN'T THE SAME ■ It's crucial to monitor your child's blood-glucose levels if she's not well, and be prepared for both too-high and too-low readings. The stress of infection, like flu, could shoot up your child's sugar numbers. But if she's vomiting, or has a poor appetite and doesn't want to eat, then her numbers can be very low. If your child is nauseous and has hypoglycemia, flat nondiet cola won't upset her stomach and will raise her blood sugar.

Children with type 1 diabetes may need insulin so they don't develop ketones in their blood, but children with type 2 don't usually face that risk, so illness is usually not as serious for them. Nonetheless, in either case, monitor frequently!

751 SICK OR WELL, TYPE 1 CHILDREN ALWAYS NEED INSULIN ■ Children who need insulin injections

always need *some* insulin—even if they're sick and not eating. Without insulin, the body breaks down its own fat, and that can lead to releasing ketones into the blood—a dangerous condition called ketoacidosis. So even when they are ill and not eating much, children with type 1 diabetes need to take insulin. How much is determined by the results of their blood-glucose readings and their pediatrician's instructions.

752 PREVENTION IS EASIER THAN TREATMENT ■ Type 2 diabetes used to be known as "adult-onset," but that

name no longer holds true, as depicted in *Time* magazine's December 8, 2003, cover story of eleven-year-old Hillary Carroll, who has "adult-onset" diabetes. Over 15 million people in the United States are affected, and as many as one third of all new cases are actually preteens and adolescents. The majority of type 2 children don't show many symptoms and may feel fine. If your child is heavy and sedentary, it may be possible to assess your child's possible risk level simply by observing his diet and activity level.

Because obese children have much more fat on their bodies, they have to produce a lot more insulin to maintain blood-glucose levels. Years of overweight can actually exhaust the insulin-producing cells that have been working so hard for so long.

753 DARK PATCHES CAN BE RED FLAGS ■ Overweight children who develop darkened and thickened patches on the skin around their armpits, waistline, or at the base of the neck need to be checked *immediately* for type 2 diabetes. This skin change is called *acanthosis nigricans,* and it's one of the few visible indications of diabetes. A urine test is inexpensive, painless, and very wise for children whose family history includes obesity or diabetes. (Alternatively, finger-stick tests can help to detect diabetes even earlier, as you don't spill glucose into urine until blood glucose is over 180 mg./dl.) So if you've scrubbed your child's "dirty neck" until it's red and it still doesn't look clean, check to see whether this skin marker is a symptom of diabetes.

754 ARE YOU SURE IT'S "JUST" BEDWETTING ■ If your child suddenly begins wetting the bed after previously being toilet-trained and dry at night, check for diabetes. While stresses from school or home or other sources can affect that behavior, bedwetting in a child who didn't have this problem before can be a symptom of diabetes—especially if the child needs to urinate frequently during the day.

755 ONE LITTLE CHANGE, OVER AND OVER, EQUALS A BIG DIFFERENCE ■ Make sure your child gets praise and encouragement for even small behavior changes because they can add up fast. Not drinking one can of soda pop can save 150 calories; giving up one can a day can add up to a fifteen-pound weight loss in a year. Make sure she knows that every bit counts!

756 IT'S A BIT LATE FOR GENES, BUT NOT TOO LATE FOR A GOOD EXAMPLE ■ The genes your child has inherited are what they are, but the lifestyle he's learning can be a major factor, too. Statistically, if both parents are overweight or have type 2 diabetes and the child is overweight, he has a 90 percent chance of developing diabetes. So family examples of exercise and moderate eating habits help more than just the one person who's exercising and eating wisely.

757 **YOUR CHILD CATCHES YOUR ATTITUDE** ■ Your behaving in matter-of-fact and unmartyred ways is vital to managing your child's diabetes. Even with an oppositional toddler, your child is learning his attitude about diabetes from watching you and your attitude.

It's also vital not to blame yourself. While you couldn't have prevented your child's condition, you *can* prevent or delay future complications by exercising care and lifestyle choices. And if your diabetic child has brothers or sisters, adopting healthy eating and exercise patterns for all of them is the best present you can give yourself and your family.

758 **DIABETES TAKES WORK AND CAREFULNESS, BUT IT'S NOT A STOPPER** ■ Children with diabetes can do anything any other child can do—except gorge on carbohydrates. Sports, hiking, bike riding, dancing—as long as the child is testing her blood-glucose levels and taking her insulin, diabetes doesn't have to stop her from any activity she did before she was diagnosed. Of course, watchfulness and monitoring are key; but careful eating and preparation before exertion can let diabetic children be kids.

759 **BE SURE YOUR CHILD'S FRIENDS KNOW IT'S NOT CATCHING** ■ Children are naturally curious, and your child's need for testing and injections will naturally raise peers' questions. Head off those questions by educating your child's friends and classmates. Most often, other children's concerns are whether they can "catch diabetes" from your child. Once information removes that worry, your child may discover that his peers are actually impressed. Depending on their ages, the rituals—doing blood tests and taking injections or using an insulin pump—or even the self-discipline involved in self-care may even elevate your child in his peers' estimation.

It shouldn't be necessary, but in this imperfect world, you may have to educate your child's friends' parents, too, that diabetes is not catching.

760

REHEARSE YOUR REACTIONS TO BAD BEHAVIOR SO THEY'RE READY WHEN YOU ARE ■ Sometimes a tantrum is just a tantrum. Sometimes it's the result of out-of-whack blood sugar. As the parent, you have the astounding 24-7 job of needing to reassert control in bad situations and, even harder, to react properly to your child's episodes of misbehavior.

This can be worlds easier if you have rehearsed your reactions mentally during calmer moments. Decide now what you would do in (a) a private or (b) a public place; whether your child needs to eat or run off some energy/has sneaked a forbidden snack/needs insulin—or is taking advantage of the situation in inconvenient but age-appropriate ways. Having a Plan A, B, C, D, and Q already formulated can save you from a great deal of guilt from having reacted in a way that you later regret.

Punishment won't change your child's blood-glucose number and so won't change the offending behavior, but a hard candy won't improve his attempts to manipulate you, either.

761

MAKE YOUR INFANT'S BED A SAFE SPACE ■ Having your infant diagnosed with diabetes can be emotionally overwhelming, but you can take some consolation and comfort in knowing that you have more help from technology and science than any parent before you. Your specialist/pediatrician can advise you about adjusting your child's insulin program around her eating patterns—not vice versa—and can also discuss using topical anesthetics to minimize the pain and fear of finger sticks.

Most important, *never* give blood-glucose tests or injections while your child is in her crib! For better sleep, feelings of security, and many other reasons, she needs to know that her bed is a "safe space."

762

IT'S ALWAYS EASIER WHEN YOU PLAY ■ A huge part of a parent's job is teaching a diabetic child self-care.

Just because it's responsible, it doesn't have to be dry or boring. Play—at your child's level—can be a wonderful teaching tool. Pretend-tests and show-me demonstrations on toys can make teaching necessary tasks more fun.

In fact, several companies even make dolls and teddy bears designed to teach children about diabetes. One such toy is Rufus, the Bear with Diabetes™, developed by a woman whose son was diagnosed with type 1 diabetes when he was three years old. (Rufus has since been joined by his sister Ruby, for little girls.)

For information on Rufus, the Bear with Diabetes™ and Ruby, the Bear with Diabetes™, contact Carol Cramer, 225 Pebble Creek Drive, Lake Zurich, IL 60047.

763 WOULDN'T IT BE GREAT TO HAVE JUST THE "CUSTOMARY" FOOD ISSUES? ■ Many toddlers have
"food issues," using not-eating as a control technique as they explore their power and development.

Your diabetic child's food issues are more immediate, with bigger stakes—but you should never let your child force you into letting her eat what she wants just because she knows you need her to eat *something*.

One technique many parents find helpful is offering limited choices among options they have preselected. Asking "Do you want oatmeal?" provokes a "No!" Asking "Do you want half an orange or half an apple?" gives your child some choice, and a feeling of power over his environment. *And* you have also gotten that healthy fruit exchange into him without a struggle or a major battle.

764 DON'T UNDERESTIMATE "MAKING MOM AND DAD HAPPY" ■ Children seek parental approval, and it's
possible to encourage their compliance without turning them into "approval junkies."

Make sure that your child receives *more* positive attention for cooperating than for rebelling. To a young child, *any* attention is welcome, regardless of whether it's positive or negative. If the volume and intensity levels go up in your home when he's *not* complying or following instructions, he'll learn how to control the household by *not* controlling his blood-glucose levels. Praise his correct behaviors and choices as specifically and as often as possible—you'll both be happier than if you yell every time something is "wrong."

765 **FEWER CHOICES MEAN LESS STRESS** ■ Take a tip from stage actors and directors: Planning and rehearsal can save you quarts of stomach acid! Predetermine and limit your child's choices for testing times, injection sites, and snacks, and present *your* predefined options as choices. Questions like "Do you want to test before or after you call Grandma for five minutes?" and "Do you want to try your right middle finger or your left one this time?" can minimize the stress involved in the procedure. These options give your child some control, and no big multiple-choice questions need to be answered.

766 **PACK YOUR PRESCHOOLER'S BACKPACK** ■ Ask the parent of almost any four- or five-year-old: That sweet little munchkin is a pure-energy machine, with completely erratic energy levels and exertion patterns. That makes preschool children especially vulnerable to hypoglycemia and all its problems and dangers. Make sure you always have protein and carbohydrate snacks or glucose tablets with you, to cover every eventuality.

767 **IT'S A NUMBER AND A CONSIDERATION—DON'T MAKE IT "GOOD" OR "BAD"** ■ Whatever numbers come up in your child's blood-glucose test results, be careful not to assign them moral values! A number isn't "good" or "bad"—it might be "higher than we'd like," or "right on target," or "a sign that we need to be more careful."

Labeling eating or test results as "good" or "bad" sets up food and esteem issues and the foundations of eating disorders that can last a lifetime.

768 **KIDS BENEFIT FROM TIGHT BLOOD-GLUCOSE CONTROL** ■ Recent research suggests that it is less risky than previously thought for children to maintain tight blood-glucose control. When older children keep their blood-glucose levels within the range that their pediatricians or endocrinologists recommend, their concentration is enhanced and their schoolwork improves.

Most doctors, however, feel that infants and toddlers benefit from a wider range of blood-glucose levels in order to prevent rapid-onset hypoglycemia and frequent trips to the emergency room. Check with your child's doctors and have them tailor the range to *your* child.

769 **YOUR DOG CAN BE YOUR FIRST ALARM** ■ Let your dog sleep in your child's bedroom. We're not copying Nana, the Saint Bernard nursemaid in *Peter Pan*, but a dog's keen sense of smell will pick up much more quickly than you can that a child with very high or very low blood sugar just smells different than usual. In fact, infants' and toddlers' wet diapers smell different to your dog, too.

When your dog wakes you in the middle of the night to take care of your diabetic child, reward it with a treat to reinforce this lifesaving behavior.

Admittedly, my evidence is anecdotal, based on stories from fellow diabetics and parents of children with diabetes. But I can tell you that my dog wakes me if my blood sugar tanks in the middle of the night. And many researchers have discovered that dogs can smell cancer, which to them apparently smells different from normal tissue.

770 **HELP YOUR CHILD WIN THE PIZZA WARS** ■ Kids love pizza, and kids with diabetes are no exception.

You don't want your child to be left out when the crowd heads for the pizzeria, but you want to protect her. The major problem is that pizza can raise blood-glucose levels for as long as forty-eight hours.

If your child has an insulin pump, ask her doctor for the proper dosage of baseline and spaced boluses to balance her high blood sugars.

Her doctor will also be able to calculate the dosage of rapid-acting and long-acting insulins if she uses insulin syringes or pens.

If your child is self-disciplined, urge her to eat only the pizza topping and maybe *only one bite of the crust.* Then she'll be able to have a marvelous time with her friends without wrecking her blood-glucose levels.

771

BIRTHDAY PARTY STRATEGIES. ■ Birthday parties, which are such happy occasions for nondiabetic children, can be frustrating events for diabetic children and their parents—especially if your little darling is popular and is invited to several parties every month.

The major problem is that so many carbohydrates are served within two or three hours—like pizza *and* birthday cake *and* ice cream *and* chips *and* pretzels.

Not letting your child go to parties is a major mistake. It isolates him, makes him unhappy and resentful, and makes him hate his disease—all guaranteed to create anything from a temper tantrum to a problem child.

Instead, work with your child's pediatrician or endocrinologist on how to balance all those carbohydrates with additional fast-acting insulin—some before the party, some several hours later or even the next day.

Depending on your child's age, intelligence, and understanding, you may be able to persuade him that the best part of the birthday cake is the cake; the icing is much too sweet and can be scraped off. The chips and pretzels can be saved for another day. Offer ice cream later in the week as a family treat.

You will probably need the experience of five or six birthday parties in order to calculate the correct amount and timing of insulin for most parties, but that's a very small price to pay for your child's enjoying all those social activities.

772

TRAIN A THIRD ADULT TO TAKE CARE OF YOUR CHILD ■ You and your spouse or partner have already been trained how to test your child's blood glucose, how to calculate her insulin requirements, how and where to inject the insulin or use a pump, how to recognize and treat hypoglycemia.

Unfortunately, that means that one of you is on 24-7 duty all the time.

Your love relationship needs some private time, too. And most parents of diabetic children discover that they haven't been able to get away for a romantic weekend since their child was first diagnosed—often several years ago. If you can train a third adult—a grandparent, relative, or close friend—to care for your child, you will be able to vacation by yourselves for at least a weekend at a time and come back relaxed and refreshed.

773 **SEND YOUR KID TO SUMMER CAMP** ■ Having diabetes does not exclude your child from summer camp, a core childhood experience. In fact, camps for diabetic kids started in the 1920s, just a few years after insulin became available. Now there are such camps in every state in the United States, every province in Canada, and in many developed countries.

Diabetic children learn a great deal from attending these special summer camps. Most importantly, they develop independence, self-confidence, athletic abilities, and comfort and knowledge that in this society—at least—*all* the kids have diabetes.

Camps have medical staffs consisting of doctors, nurses, and dietitians. The counselor-camper ratio is high, and counselors are trained and experienced in reacting to potential blood-glucose difficulties.

There are day camps for younger children and sleepaway camps for older ones (usually ages 7–17). Some camps offer family programs, and many camps provide partial or full scholarships, depending on need.

When choosing a camp for your child, make sure that the medical staff checks all campers during the night to detect and correct any blood-glucose problems.

774 **WALK YOUR CHILD TO SCHOOL** ■ Walking your child to school gives both of you some more exercise. It's also a wonderful opportunity for serious or playful one-on-one discussions.

775 **PRAISE YOUR CHILD'S *OTHER* ACHIEVEMENTS** ■ Is your child gifted academically? Musically? Athletically? Has he or she earned badges in the Boy or Girl Scouts? Been elected to class office?

Emphasize *these* achievements over those related to diabetes and blood-glucose control. Concentrate on the *rest* of your child's life, not on the diabetic part, which already receives a lot of attention.

776 **QUESTION THAT SQUIRMING** ■ If your school-age daughter squirms a lot in her chair, ask if she's "itchy in private places." The sugar that spills over into diabetics' urine makes girls more susceptible to urinary tract and vaginal infections. If she seems to have a recurrence of such problems, no matter how young she is, have her blood-glucose levels checked.

777 **MAKE SURE THE TEACHER AND SCHOOL KNOW WHAT'S REQUIRED** ■ The Individuals with Disabilities Education Act (IDEA) and Section 504 of the Rehabilitation Act of 1973 both protect children who have diabetes against discrimination. They are supposed to ensure that all children can take part in all school activities, and still handle their medical needs. If your child's school program doesn't make the necessary provisions, take the attitude that they need educating, and do it gently. Indignation—even righteous indignation—will make opponents of the very people whose assistance you'll need.

778 **NOT EVERY INDIVIDUALIZED EDUCATION PROGRAM IS FOR SPECIAL ED** ■ Every school that receives federal funding must comply with the Individuals with Disabilities Education Act (IDEA). That means you can request an Individual Education Program (IEP) and a Section 504 Accommodation for your child, and the school must meet with you about your child's special needs. The School Bill of Rights for Children with Diabetes includes a list of services. Look it up online, so you don't miss anything that could assist your child.

779
WHERE TO BEGIN WHEN TALKING TO OPPOSING FORCES ■ Most schools are clear on their responsibilities to children with diabetes, as per the Individuals with Disabilities Education Act (IDEA), which guarantees that your child can care for his diabetes while in school. Many school systems can no longer afford full-time school nurses, but they are required to allow your child time and opportunity for blood-glucose self-testing, unrestricted access to drinking water and the bathroom, snacks as needed, participation in gym classes and field trips, and the privacy and opportunity to inject insulin when necessary.

If your child's school refuses to comply, your first step should be to file a complaint with your state's department of education.

780
INFORM YOURSELF BEFORE TAKING ON THE BOARD OF EDUCATION ■ The National Information Center for Children and Youth with Disabilities (NICHCY) is a government-sponsored information clearinghouse that also covers obtaining assistance at school, including the names and contact information for state officials and education departments.

The National Information Center for Children and Youth
   with Disabilities (NICHCY)
P.O. Box 1492
Washington, DC 20013
Phone: (800) 695-0285
Fax: (202) 884-8441
nichcy@aed.org
www.nichcy.org

781
THE FLIP SIDE OF PRIVILEGE IS RESPONSIBILITY ■ Your child must be permitted to bring syringes to

school if she injects insulin, but she also needs to be responsible about their disposal after use. Your prenotification of the school's officials—plus your child's responsible behavior regarding syringes' use and disposal—will distinguish her "needles" from any of the administration's fears about "drug paraphernalia."

782

ASSUME THEY'RE MISINFORMED, RATHER THAN INSENSITIVE MORONS ■ If your child's school administration isn't cooperative about the special needs of his diabetes, be as gracious as possible for as long as you can before invoking the legal system. The U.S. Department of Health and Human Services publishes the booklet, "How to File a Complaint with the Office of Civil Rights Under Section 504." Your child's medical condition mandates nondiscriminatory treatment—but exhaust all other possibilities before making a literal federal case of it. Be aware that filing a complaint is the first step to litigation, which could cause your child some day-to-day friction at school with administrators, teachers, or smart-mouthed peers.

783

"FAIR" IS ABOUT EVERYONE GETTING WHAT THEY NEED ■ Children have innate fairness-sensing mechanisms, and some are not above using claims of perceived unfairness as a manipulation tool. Your child's individual snacks or extra bathroom privileges may be what's inspiring any jealousy from other students. Should she run into classmate complaints about her "extra privileges," don't burden her self-esteem further by trying to "even up the score" by pointing out the disadvantages of her condition. Instead, instruct your child to tell bullies and teases that "fair" means everybody gets what they need, and not everybody needs the same thing.

784

ONE PAGE IS BEST, FOR BOTH RÉSUMÉS AND INSTRUCTIONS ■ Most children's special diabetic needs during school can be listed, double-spaced, on one page. Giving your child's teacher a single sheet makes it easy to read, post, and reread in a rushed or worried moment, and copies can easily be placed with the school's principal, nurse, and secretaries.

Make it as easy as possible for others to assist your child. Your goal is to transmit all necessary information in a way that's as simple and unintimidating as possible.

785 TIMING IS EVERYTHING, AND NOT JUST FOR INSULIN ■ Choose your time carefully for speaking to your child's teacher. Trying to snag her attention when you're dropping off your child is a bad way to begin that relationship. Once classtime starts, it's unfair to distract her from her primary responsibilities, even "just for a minute," and will give you a much less interested listener.

Much better plan: Call the school—before the academic year begins, if possible—and ask for a brief meeting with the teacher and the principal, so everybody can get onto the same page at a time when your child's welfare is the only topic of discussion.

786 THAT IMPORTANT ID BRACELET . . . ■ If your child goes to school—even preschool—he needs a medical ID bracelet marked "DIABETIC." Make sure he puts it on every day when he gets dressed. (You may have to remove a few links so that it will fit snugly and won't fall off.)

787 . . . AND WATCH ■ As a mark of his being grown up enough to go to school, give your child an inexpensive watch and teach him to tell time. That way he can judge when to check his blood glucose, or when to have a snack.

788 EARLY PUBERTY CAN CAUSE BLOOD-GLUCOSE PROBLEMS ■ In the past fifty years, puberty has come earlier and earlier. In the 1950s, it used to begin around the age of thirteen; now it often begins as early as age nine or ten.

When you notice the beginning signs of puberty in your child, brace yourself for the inevitable: your child's rapidly changing body and outrageous mood swings, caused by surging new hormones.

While all of these changes are true for all adolescents and their parents, they affect children with diabetes and their parents especially hard. Diabetic kids can experience wildly fluctuating blood sugars, so ask your pediatrician or endocrinologist to double their test-strip prescriptions so your child can test every few hours, if necessary.

Be aware that puberty can also trigger type 2 diabetes in children who are seriously overweight. If your child is overweight, make sure that a blood-glucose test is part of every medical examination.

789 **TEACH YOUR CHILD BODY CONFIDENCE** ■ Fact: Most children are not thin enough or beautiful enough to be magazine models, just as 99.9999 percent of adults are not.

Start teaching your child very early to be happy about her body, even if she's a little overweight. You do not want her to practice bulimia or starvation as a dieting tool, even if all her friends are doing it.

Take the opportunity to show your daughter some of the legendary nude paintings by Rubens, Rembrandt, and Renoir to teach her that physical beauty and confidence come in all sizes and shapes. At the same time, encourage her to eat sensibly and be physically active.

Note: Although girls predominate, recent research shows that teenage boys have been going on starvation diets and practicing bulimia, too.

790 **MAKE GROCERY SHOPPING A LEARNING EXPERIENCE** ... ■ Even preschoolers with diabetes can learn a lot about nutrition and making healthy choices during a trip to the supermarket. Involve them in making decisions—you can limit their options—and respect their food likes and dislikes. (Don't be surprised if they change next month.)

Older children and adolescents can add to their skills, learning how to choose produce, meat, and fish, how to read and interpret labels, how to work within a food budget, and how each choice that is made impacts other choices.

791 **. . . AND COOKING, TOO** ■ Even young children can help in the kitchen—they love to! Preschoolers can help make salads, knead and punch down bread, and stir ingredients in a bowl. Older children can learn to use knives (carefully, under supervision!) and stovetops and ovens (ditto!) Consult with them on trying out new recipes, tweaking old favorites, and even creating new dishes—for example, starting with chicken, adding which vegetables, herbs, spices.

792 **TRY A MINITRIATHLON** ■ Scale down a triathlon for your child. (It will still be exciting and pleasurable; remember to test blood glucose first and have a snack, if needed.)

Younger children can probably ride their bicycles up and down the street once, walk or run the same distance, and swim two laps freestyle in the backyard pool. Teenagers can multiply these distances by five times, then ten.

Reward your child for finishing the triathlon—don't time kids until they ask you to. Considering their exertion, ice cream is a wonderfully suitable reward.

793 **HOW MUCH SLACK CAN YOU CUT YOUR TEEN?** ■ Physicians, psychologists, and diabetics can all testify: Going through puberty as a diabetic is infinitely more complicated than dealing with either situation alone. The mood swings and raging hormones of adolescence are multiplied, warped, and amplified by the mood swings and raging hormones of galloping blood-glucose levels, and the disease is a perfect setup for teenage risk-taking behavior. As much as possible, help your teen keep social and personal identity issues separate from diabetic issues. Blood-glucose-control battles and even some safety issues need to be seen by parents through the age-normal prisms of independence struggles and autonomy issues.

794 **PLAN NOW FOR THOSE TEEN YEARS** ■ Without putting too Pollyanna-ish a face on the situation, I think that parents whose young children are diagnosed with type 1 or type 2 diabetes are oddly lucky in one respect: They can establish habits, expectations, and influence from the child's early age, and this can be much easier than presenting new restrictions to a headstrong teen. The openness, respect, and authority you establish with your toddler or school-age child will assist you both greatly when he reaches his midteens.

795 **THE SKIN THEY'RE IN CAN BE MORE COMFORTABLE** ■ Your child's objections to being diabetic are based largely on the dietary restrictions and discomforts of the condition. Nothing else is really real to him, and future complications seem forever away, if he even believes they are possible.

Minimizing comfort complaints can make your child's diabetes much easier emotionally as well as physically. For dry skin problems, especially in winter, moisturizing lotions like Jergens, Curel, Vaseline Intensive Care and others can help, but some children may need stronger remedies. Look for body lotions without alcohol (it's drying), and mineral oil because of its properties as a moisture sealant. Ask your pharmacist or health-food store for Bag Balm, a cream invented for healing cows' udders. It also turns out to be fabulous on skiers' frostbitten and windburned faces, and many nurses have quietly used it for years to prevent bedsores on their patients. As Bag Balm has the consistency of petroleum jelly and a strong smell, give your child enough time for it to be absorbed and the smell to dissipate before getting dressed.

796 **DON'T LET A LABEL THROW YOU—OR THEM** ■ From kindergarten until long past our teen years, a label can rankle and plow up all kinds of negative feelings. Try to remember, and instill in your child: Attitudes hold you back. Because some federal laws label diabetes as a "disability," diabetic children are entitled to

special considerations in schools: everything from "shadow teachers" for children whose blood-glucose swings cause behavior problems to extra time and assistance when taking the SAT tests. More than any other sensitive child, yours needs to learn that a label is "just a word, not a sentence."

797

WE'RE FROM THE GOVERNMENT AND WE'RE HERE TO HELP YOU ■ The National Diabetes Education Program has information on assisting children with diabetes. Its Resources on Diabetes in Children and Adolescents offers a booklet titled "Helping the Student with Diabetes Succeed. A Guide for School Personnel." It's invaluable for parents, in order to know what educators and administrators should know. The booklet is free and is available from the NDEP Web site, http://ndep.nih.gov.

Another arm of the federal government, the Department of Justice's Civil Rights Division, has details of the Americans with Disabilities Act and what to do about discrimination. Log on to http://www.susdoj.gov/disabilities.htm.

798

DON'T BE INTIMIDATED, HERE'S A GOOD PLACE TO START ■ If you've already Google'd "diabetes," you've already been swamped with way too much information. Don't be alarmed. The National Diabetes Information Clearinghouse (NDIC) breaks a lot of data and resources into accessible chunks. They'll answer questions about diabetes by phone, fax, mail, and e-mail; just remember to call between 8:30 AM and 5:00 PM Eastern Time, Monday through Friday.

The NDIC offers booklets, brochures, and online information, copyright-free and on several reading levels. The Web site can also refer you to local health organizations. Contact the NDIC at:

National Diabetes Information Clearinghouse
One Information Way
Bethesda, MD 20892-3560
Phone: (800) 860-8747 or (301) 654-3327

Fax: (301) 907-8906
E-mail: ndic@info.niddk.nih.gov

799 OPEN WIDE AND SAY "AAAH" ■ Tooth and gum problems can be more prevalent in diabetics. Everyone's plaque buildup includes germs, but high blood glucose helps germs and bacteria flourish and multiply. That leads to bad breath and sore and swollen gums that bleed when you brush your teeth.

Children with diabetes can have tooth and gum problems more often if their blood glucose stays high. Check your child's smile regularly. Sore, bleeding gums are the first signs of periodontal (gum) disease, which can lead to infection in the gums and bone that holds the teeth. Infection may cause your child's gums to pull away from his teeth, and could even lead to premature tooth loss.

800 MAKE SURE YOUR CHILD'S A SHOE-IN ■ Foot damage is a constant threat to diabetics, who may not feel blisters or injuries when they happen. Make sure your child always wears socks or stockings with her shoes or slippers, to avoid blisters. Knee-high stockings or socks that are too tight at the top are also an invitation to problems because they restrict circulation.

Most importantly, check your child's shoes weekly to make sure that they still fit well. Make sure that a growth spurt isn't trapping your child's feet in suddenly-too-small shoes. Do your shoe-shopping at the end of the day, when your child's feet are at their biggest. And have your child break in new shoes by wearing them only for an hour or two a day for the first week.

801 CHECK YOUR CHILD'S SHOES EVERY MORNING ■ Everyone in Texas and the Southwest learns to check inside a shoe before putting it on—scorpions, spiders, and other nasty critters may have crawled into the warm, dark recess. But even in Saskatchewan or Duluth, checking inside your child's shoes before putting them on is a good habit to develop: Small toys, loosened shoe tacks, or other sharp-edged hazards might be hiding, ready to injure your child's feet.

802 **DON'T PUSH FOOD ON YOUR KIDS** ■ Even toddlers and preschoolers are much better at gauging their appetites than their parents are. Your kids are more likely not to overeat if you let them serve themselves or if you serve them small portions and let *them* ask for more.

Urging them to take one more spoonful for Mommy/Daddy/Grandma and the whole family tree can lead to lifelong overeating and childhood obesity.

803 **MAKE SURE YOUR PEDIATRICIAN CHECKS YOUR CHILD'S BLOOD PRESSURE** ■ Pediatricians should be taking blood-pressure readings at every routine visit starting at *age three*. High blood pressure can start in children and do great damage before it is officially diagnosed or treated, and children with diabetes are especially vulnerable. Ask the doctor to check your child's blood pressure at least during the annual checkup.

804 **HAVE YOUR CHILD CHECKED FOR GLUTEN SENSITIVITY** ■ Medical researchers now recommend that children with type 1 diabetes be tested for celiac disease, or gluten sensitivity. Celiac disease is a genetic disorder that makes people unable to tolerate gluten, a protein found in wheat, rye, and barley. When they eat foods containing gluten, their immune system responds by damaging the lining of the small intestine. Since the damaged areas can't absorb nutrients properly, people with celiac disease become malnourished—no matter how much or how well they eat. Controlling your child's glucose levels and nutritional intake will be much easier when you know whether she has a gluten sensitivity.

805 MAKE YOUR RELATIONSHIP HEALTHY ■ Having a child with diabetes means even more riding herd, questioning and checking, and striving for control from parents. Keeping that need for strict control must be confined to the disease, without overbalancing the rest of your relationship with your child. Maintaining a healthy relationship with your child demands a great deal of self-control and self-awareness on your part. If necessary, keep an actual private count of your positive interactions each day. Make sure that you're not just a cop or a "measurer," but also a warm, safe, nurturing parent. If most of your conversations with your child are about restrictions or control, expect power struggles and resentment.

806 DON'T PUNISH FOR DIABETES-RELATED SLIPS ■ "Discipline" actually means "guidance." Punishing your child for anything relating to his diabetes makes the disease seem even more unfair. All kids sneak sweets; when yours does, too, receiving the same punishment as when he does something deliberate or defiant makes having the disease feel even harder.

Yes, the results are worse for your child, but it's also true that kids forget and accidents happen. If you can, use diabetes-related slips and sneaks as teaching moments, rather than punishment occasions. Your getting angry can inspire equal and opposing anger, or hopelessness or guilt—or all of these emotions.

807 YOUR CHILD IS A SEPARATE PERSON, AND NOBODY'S ALWAYS PERFECT ■ Two of the biggest stress-inducers in parents are (wrongly) seeing their children as extensions of themselves rather than as separate individuals, and (wrongly) seeing diabetes as a flaw or a failure. Before you laugh, ask yourself if you've ever uttered the phrase, "How could a child of mine . . . ?"

Diabetes is a physical condition, not a failure; and your child's physiology does not reflect on your character or parenting. Don't add guilt or pride to the already-stressful mix of emotions; instead, use that energy to assist your child in finding coping strategies.

808 **ARE YOUR CHILD'S SLIPUPS ACCIDENTS, OR A CONTROL STRUGGLE?** ■ Occasionally forgetting his diabetes paraphernalia or insulin is one thing; habitual problems are something else. Make sure that the consequences of poor diabetes choices are appropriate to the "crime," and instruct your child on better choices. Almost all children want more freedom; taking some away when it's misused is much more effective—and instructive—than almost any other punishment.

809 **PLAN AHEAD, SO YOUR EMOTIONAL ARMOR IS UP WHEN YOU NEED IT** ■ People with diabetes can't always be held accountable for their actions when their blood glucose is low. As much as words or blows can hurt, remember that children with diabetes aren't in their usual mental or emotional states when their glucose levels are too low. As difficult as it is for you to hear or get through, it's vital to remember that your child may be speaking or acting in ways that she may not even remember later. Plan now, so you'll be able to remember then, that these things wouldn't happen if she were in normal range.

810 **PARENTS AREN'T ALWAYS EQUAL PARTNERS** ■ It can be hard to raise a diabetic child, and two-parent families aren't always equal-load carriers. Frequently, one parent carries more of the workload of the child's diabetes care; even more frequently, one parent carries more of the emotional load.

If you are the "less-burdened" parent, try to determine the scheduling limitations or discomfort with your child's illness—whatever keeps you less involved. If you are the parent who carries more of the load, do all you can to bring your spouse more into the picture. Understanding that diabetes is not a failure or imperfection gives you more insight into how it affects you, your spouse, and your child's life. Make efforts to minimize resentments so that you don't alienate your child from either parent.

811 **TRADE FOR TREATS** ■ Yes, the possible dire consequences may be the first thing that occurs to you when you catch your child sneaking sweets; but teaching your child to "trade for treats" is much more useful, in both the long term and the immediate moment.

Preteens aren't too young to learn how to compensate for treats. If he understands the balancing of food with insulin, and knows to tell an adult when he's hungry or having cravings, both of you will be happier. You'll worry less about the possible consequences of his sneaking food, and he'll be more at ease knowing that he has a loving, caring backup. Teach him early: Never, never sneak food without letting a parent or teacher know.

812 **WHAT TO SAY TO MAKE EVERYTHING WORSE** ■ Women are rightly offended when someone suggests that their emotional state is due to monthly hormone fluctuations. Diabetics can often be just as offended when asked if their behavior is due to low blood sugar. Even when your intentions are good, tendering that question is likely to infuriate someone who's already upset or angry—especially if you're right!

Rather than inquiring about a blood-glucose level, consider offering your child a multiple choice: "Can I get you some turkey or a banana or something, as long as I'm up?" Phrased that way, a solution is possible without triggering emotional oversensitivity—or invalidating a real feeling by ascribing it to hormones. Your child could actually be justifiably angry without being hypoglycemic!

813 **DON'T CALL YOUR CHILD BY HIS DISEASE** ■ Let your child keep his personhood and not be labeled by his disease. Whenever possible, refer to him as "Joey, a person with diabetes," rather than "a diabetic."

814

IF POSSIBLE, HAVE THE BABYSITTER TAKE A RED CROSS COURSE ■ The best babysitter isn't just someone your child likes who's free on Saturday night. As your child needs special attention regarding when and what she eats, your babysitter needs some educating about the symptoms of low blood sugar and how to treat it. You'll have to do much of this individual educating yourself.

For the general, nondiabetic babysitting issues, the American Red Cross has developed an excellent course in babysitting geared to teenagers, and your local chapter can tell you if this course is offered near you. Safe Sitter is another organization that offers a babysitting course. Call (800) 255-4089 to see if there is a program near you.

815

MAKE YOUR CHILD A CARD-CARRYING DIABETIC ■ Teaching your child to take ownership of her diabetes is vital: Who will be watching her once she leaves your home? Joining the American Diabetes Association and the Juvenile Diabetes Foundation makes great sense for anyone with diabetes in the family. Memberships offer many benefits not listed in their pamphlets. Your child can read about diabetes in materials appropriate to her age level, making self-care easier and taking some of the burden off you, the parent.

816

SCHOOL LUNCHES AS PORTABLE SMORGASBORDS GET EATEN MORE ■ Prepackaged lunch kits are available in combinations suitable for diabetic meal plans, but read the labels carefully: They're loaded with MSG, fat, and salt. More importantly, you can't supervise the quality of the ingredients.

Making your own lunch kits, using little plastic containers, lets you duplicate the appeal of the commercial packs—and still control what's going into the lunch. Cubes of grilled chicken or low-fat cheese, plus baby carrots, cherry tomatoes, and berries, each in its own small plastic tub, turns a healthy lunch into a scavenger hunt. Opening each little case makes discovering the next treat fun, and having small quantities of many foods increases the likelihood that your child will eat enough of the right things.

817 **COVER YOUR CHILD'S HEALTH WHILE TRAVELING** ■ You may go on vacation, but your child's diabetes won't be going on hold. Check with your health insurance company to make sure you and your child will be covered wherever you travel. If not, look into a special insurance policy for your vacation.

Talk to your child's doctor before you leave, especially if you're going out of the country or even to another time zone; you'll need adjustments in her insulin or medication schedule. Also, make sure her shots are up to date, and provide her with emergency medical ID and information.

And always carry twice as much insulin or medication as your child would normally need for the time away. *Don't pack it in your suitcase—put it in your carry-on bag.*

818 **PLAN FOR WINTER** ■ Children with diabetes need to do some extra planning for winter. The drier air can make or worsen skin problems and itches, and winter also brings more colds and flu. Be forewarned: Illness stresses the body, so blood-glucose levels go up when your child is ill, making it harder to control his diabetes. Talk to your child's endocrinologist or pediatrician now about how to handle sick days.

819 **CONSIDER SEWING SOLUTIONS FOR CHILDREN ON PUMPS** ■ A needle and thread and a little creativity can make it easier for your child to wear an insulin pump. Even very young children are using insulin pumps now, but toddlers' clothes frequently don't have the belts and design features that allow the pump to be worn easily. If your child resists the harness that comes with some pumps, make her a new undergarment: Sewing a square of cotton jersey (from an outgrown T-shirt?) onto the back of her T-shirt creates a pouch that holds a pump easily. And her remodeled T-shirt needs no special laundering instructions. She can wear the shirt under other clothes, and putting the pouch in the back takes it out of her way but still leaves it accessible.

820 **MOM WAS RIGHT: BREAKFAST IS THE MOST IMPORTANT MEAL** ■ We've all heard that breakfast is the most important meal of the day. That's even more true for children with diabetes. Your child will need food for energy to start his day. Blood sugars may be low after not having eaten all night, and a good breakfast of foods on his meal plan will help him think and feel better.

One note: An egg would seem to be an obvious protein choice, but research shows that egg yolks may not be good for people with diabetes, especially if their cholesterol is high. Instead, consider cooking liquid egg substitute, or serving low-fat cottage cheese or string cheese, Canadian bacon or lean ham, sliced turkey or lean roast beef, water-pack tuna, a handful of nuts, or peanut butter.

821 **BE SAFE TO TALK TO** ■ Children need to feel safe to talk about their diabetes and how it makes them feel. Difficult as it may be, separating your feelings from just listening is vital. As a beloved grown-up, you are not only a source of information, you also need to be a safe harbor for frustrations and fears about the repercussions of ignoring diabetes. Don't make your responses make your child equate a high blood-glucose level with shame and blame—he needs you to be safe to talk to—about *anything*.

822 **DON'T NEGLECT YOUR OTHER CHILDREN** ■ This should be obvious. (Nobody said it was easy!) 'Nuff said.

8

Tips from Diabetics Who Live Alone

ALL THE TIPS in this chapter relate to feeling—and being—less vulnerable and less prone to accidents even though you have diabetes and live alone. When you feel safe, you are less stressed. As a result, your blood-glucose levels stay more even.

823 **CELEBRATE YOUR SINGLENESS** ■ Attitude can be everything, especially when you're the only one in the house. Yes, living alone has the drawback of occasional loneliness; it also has the advantage of enormous privacy. You can run around the house in a moose mask all day if you like (and if the curtains are closed). You can watch TV at 2:00 AM, grill a hamburger for breakfast, or do yoga in the living room in the nude. Since everything in life is a trade, focus on what you gain by your single lifestyle, rather than griping about what you may feel is lacking in any one moment.

824 **DON'T LEAVE TOWN WITHOUT IT** ■ Don't even think of going out of town without giving a trusted friend a copy of your itinerary. Every single person should do this, diabetic or not. If you haven't alerted people to expect you at a certain place at a certain time, how could they know if something were amiss? Doing this assists you and gives peace of mind to everyone who cares about you.

825 IS THAT YOUR WATCH VIBRATING, OR ARE YOU JUST GLAD TO SEE ME? ■ Self-care for your diabetes is your responsibility, but living alone makes it that much more important to remember all the checkpoints in your day. A fabulous but subtle helper is a vibrating watch: Rather than sounding an alarm, it gives the wearer an unmistakable (but silent) wake-up or reminder. Unless you're holding someone's hand at the moment, the shaking is your own private alert. Originally created for people with hearing loss, a vibrating watch can keep us diabetics on schedule, too. Go online and Google "vibrating watch"; you'll find an extensive assortment of makes and prices to choose from.

826 GIVE YOURSELF A FREE SPACE ■ One of the roughest aspects of living alone is misplacing something vital. You pretty much need your glasses to find your glasses, and where are you if you can't find your car keys?

Designate a spot in your home—the bottom of your underwear drawer, a kitchen shelf, next to the bathroom sink, whatever—to be the "home base" for possessions that you absolutely *can't* lose. When your glasses aren't on the bridge of your nose, they'll be in your "spot." When your car keys aren't in your hand or in the ignition, they'll be in your "spot." Be as obsessive and compulsive about this as possible— you'll never be sorry.

You may want another space—near your bed?—for your glucose meter, test strips, and glucose tablets.

827 KNOW YOUR NEIGHBORS ■ Because you live alone, get to know your neighbors. Be aware of who their family and relatives are, and get an idea of their normal schedules. Preventing a burglary next door may keep you safe as well.

Also, tell your neighbors that you have diabetes, and tell them what to do if they don't see you at the usual times.

828 **KNOCK THREE TIMES** ■ If you live in an apartment or town house where you share a common wall with a neighbor, arrange a signal in case you need help.

829 **TAKE YOUR DIABETES TO SEA** ■ Who says controlling your diabetes can't be fun? Go online and see how many different cruises are offered for people with diabetes. Not only would you be aboard a ship with like-minded cruising companions, you'd also be catered to by chefs cooking for your special needs.

And check with your tax consultant: Some special-for-diabetics cruises also offer educational seminars aboard. See whether you can write off a portion of the cost of your vacation, since it *is* medically oriented . . .

830 **YOU KNOW HOW TO WHISTLE, DON'T YOU?** ■ Put a whistle on your keychain, and consider wearing one on a ribbon or chain around your neck—outside and inside the house. If you're outside and someone approaches to bother you, blowing that whistle makes you too much audible trouble to mess with. And just as important, wearing your whistle *inside* your house lets you summon help—sometimes even through apartment walls! It doesn't have to be an expensive stainless-steel coach's whistle—often plastic dime-store whistles can emit loud, piercing shrieks, and come in bright neon colors that are easy to spot at the bottom of a handbag.

831 **DAWDLE OVER DINNER** ■ Too many people who live alone race through their meals in front of the TV. Make your dinner last at least forty-five minutes. When you slow down, some wonderful things happen:

▶ You turn eating into dining, a pleasurable experience.

▶ You give your body the chance to start feeling full, a process that takes twenty to thirty minutes.

▶ And this means that you won't overeat mindlessly, when you really don't want to.

832 **USE A BUDDY SYSTEM** ■ You should have someone to check in with every morning. Your buddy doesn't have to be a fellow diabetic; anyone who lives alone and might need help will benefit from the arrangement, and so will you.

Your call can be brief: "Hi, it's me. Are you OK? I'm OK. Do you need anything?"

What counts is that you have both made sure that your friend is alive and well.

833 **DON'T BE TOO PROUD TO USE A CANE** ■ Many people use a cane in the winter to navigate snowy and icy streets, only because they can't afford to risk breaking a bone. If you have diabetes, your balance may be compromised, so this is even more important for you. One of my neighbors, who does not have diabetes, took a fall on New Year's Day and wound up with a compound shoulder fracture that necessitated hours of surgery and months of physical therapy!

Use a cane that's beautiful so that it will give you pleasure. Mine has a brass dog's head, and I'm looking for others so that they become fashion statements. If you live alone where there is a lot of snow or ice, ski poles and/or crampons may help you avoid a fall.

834 **MAYBE YOU SHOULDN'T LOCK UP** ■ Admittedly, this advice is debatable. It depends on how safe your home and neighborhood are. It comes from a friend who has severe diabetes and who averages two or three trips to the emergency room every year. While he is glad that he's been rescued in time, he has gotten tired of EMS technicians breaking down his door to reach him.

If you feel safe in your home or apartment, keep your door *unlocked* when you go to sleep. If you need an ambulance for an emergency, EMS personnel won't have to break down your door—and then leave it open.

835 **DON'T BE SHY ■** If you live in an apartment, let your building staff know that you have diabetes and what your schedule is.

Leave standing instructions that if they don't see you by a certain time every morning, to ring your bell and—if there is no answer—to call 911.

836 **BATHROOM SMARTS I: GET THE RIGHT GRAB RAILS ■** Install heavy-duty grab rails in the bathtub. Make sure they will bear *at least 100 pounds more than your weight;* anything less is risky.

837 **BATHROOM SMARTS II: CREATE A SKIDPROOF TUB ■** Cover your tub with attractive adhesive motifs. Get these grippers as large as possible so that your feet will fit completely on them.

838 **BATHROOM SMARTS III: THE RIGHT PHONE ■** Cordless phones are usually the first phones people think of because they are so portable. But for bathroom (and bedside) I recommend a phone that is directly connected to the circuitry because they will usually work even during power failures. In fact, during the Great Blackout of August 14–15, 2003, only my bedroom phone, which was hard-wired into the circuitry, worked. The five or six cordless and cell phones in different parts of the apartment were completely nonfunctioning!

839 USE YOUR PRIVACY TO CREATE NEW HABITS ■ Habits often make us what we are; in fact, longtime ingrained habits are likely what make controlling blood-glucose levels so difficult. But behavior experts say that creating a new habit can be done in just twenty-eight days—that's less than a month!

So, since one of the joys of living alone is the privacy, use it! Put up big signs in the kitchen, or by the television, reminding yourself of your new goals. And make some healthier new habits, so that doing what comes naturally—by unthinking routine—improves your life.

840 OUTWIT THE PORTION-CONTROL MARKETERS ■ Almost everything you buy is sized wrong: Bottles, bags, boxes almost always contain at least two portions—usually more. Make unpacking your groceries a two-step process. Before putting away purchases, break them down into portion-sized servings. Zipper-lock plastic bags make this very easy to do, so that grabbing a measured portion becomes effortless. It's the simplest way not to "just eat the broken chips" or "just finish the carton" or "polish off the rest of the bottle."

841 A COOKBOOK FOR SINGLE DIABETICS ■ The advantage of cooking for yourself is knowing the purity and quality of the ingredients, knowing what went into what's going on your plate. A book by two registered dietitians, Kathleen Stanley and Connie Crawley, offers more than 100 recipes for breakfasts, lunches, dinners, and snacks for diabetics who are cooking single portions. *Quick & Easy Diabetic Recipes for One* is available at most brick-and-mortar and online bookstores, or through the American Diabetes Association.

842 PREPARE NOW FOR THE URGE TO GRAB SOMETHING ■ Alone in the house, with nothing tasty-and-permissible ready to eat, is almost a slam-dunk setup to grab something quick-and-easy—and off your eating plan. You can avoid this by doing a little preparation at a time when you're well-fed and in no hurry: Grill and wrap up a chicken breast, cut and clean some veggies, and make sure you have something immediately grabbable and satisfying. Even a can of chickpeas provides a complete protein with complex carbohydrates that provides a lot of chewing satisfaction.

843 **BE A CARD-CARRYING PERSON WITH DIABETES ■** Your just-in-case scenario should include at least a what-if contingency, in case you were ever unable to speak for yourself. Wearing a medical ID bracelet and carrying a card in your wallet next to your driver's license is more than smart, it's vital. If your commuter train got derailed or a truck ran a light and plowed into your car, giving emergency personnel as much information as possible about your body will let them save valuable time and get you better care.

844 **CELL PHONES WERE INVENTED JUST FOR YOU ■** The cliché "I've fallen and I can't get up" became a cliché because it's true so often—and not just for senior citizens. Living alone means nobody else there, and the flip side of that freedom and peace is no help if you *do* need help. Today's size, affordability, and availability of cell phones means that living alone isn't as dangerous anymore. A little device half the size and weight of your hand can fit in any pocket and follow you from room to room in your house. If you don't already have a cell phone, get one now.

845 **STAY MOTIVATED ■** Living alone means it's often hard to stay motivated about tight blood-glucose control, keeping spirits up during downturns in life events, and other problems. Keep pets, pictures of loved ones, or even portraits of heroes and heroines around in full view. They can serve as reminders of love and courage during bad or just lonely times. Take strength from the knowledge that others depend on you to do the right thing, and if nobody currently does, then motivate yourself with the knowledge that you're behaving in ways that would make your heroes proud of you.

846 **HIGH-TECH HELPERS** ■ "I forgot" just isn't an excuse that holds water anymore, ever since PDAs began including health-tracking software. Palm Pilots, Handspring Visors, and other PDAs have become affordable, and commercial and even some free software is now available to track all aspects of diabetes management from the palm of your hand. And ladies, if you're looking for a gift for a guy with diabetes, gadgets with bells and whistles can make even self-testing fun!

847 **YOU DESERVE A FIRE EXTINGUISHER OF YOUR OWN** ■ Living alone means being the strongest link in your own chain—but also the weakest. Be prepared to handle any situation on your own by laying in the supplies you might need in an emergency. Put a small fire extinguisher in your kitchen and a second one in your bedroom. And check the batteries in your smoke alarm twice a year!

848 **PREPARE TO TAKE ON MOTHER NATURE SINGLE-HANDEDLY** ■ If you live in an area prone to earthquakes, tornadoes, or ice storms, build a preparedness kit with a flashlight, some cash in case the ATMs are down, sneakers, deck shoes, or lightweight hiking boots, a Mylar blanket in case the heat goes out, extra socks and gloves, and a spare pair of glasses. More importantly, you should also put by three days' worth of provisions and medications so you can get along until rescue workers can reach you or restore the utilities.

849 **LIVING ALONE SAFELY WITH "BRUNO"** ■ Living alone means quiet and peace whenever you want it, but you might not want strangers to know it's just you behind that door with the hardware-store lock. Consider posting a second name on your mailbox, something that sounds tough-but-not-made-up macho. That way, deliverymen and strangers casing your home will have to speculate on dealing with you *and* "Bruno McCormick"—not just you, alone.

850
LICENSED CONTRACTORS ARE MORE THAN WORTH IT ■ Living alone means never hiring an unlicensed contractor to work in or even outside your home—even if your best friend swears by him. Contractors' licenses are overseen by local or state boards (depends on your municipality), which prefer to discipline their own from within. Hiring unlicensed people to do repairs or chores might sound cheaper, but your risks are higher—and not just financially.

851
CHEAP AND CHEERFUL EARLY WARNINGS ■ Unless you have a cat, hanging inexpensive glass wind chimes on your doorknob when you lock up for the night can be a life-saver: If you hear them tinkling in the night, somebody is trying your door. Little bells would work as well unless, again, you have a cat that would love to bat it around in play.

Hearing the wind chimes jingle gives you time to dial up 911 on your bedside phone. You *do* have a phone at your bedside, right? And some people go as far as putting bottles or other breakables on their windowsills, easy to hear if someone tries to break in.

852
DON'T DISMISS YOUR INSTINCTS ■ Whenever you feel uneasy being alone, trust your instincts. One crime-prevention expert put it best: "We are the only mammal on the planet that dismisses our instinct most of the time," usually out of concern about overdramatizing or being seen as hysterical or paranoid.

If you sense you're being followed, go inside a business or store and ask to call 911. If someone is approaching you, cross the street. If you are cornered, scream and holler and call attention to yourself—be more trouble to bother than you're worth.

853
KEEP A FLASHLIGHT IN OR NEAR YOUR BED ■ There are lots of reasons to keep this handy little tool nearby: to check on suspicious noises, to light your way during a power failure,

even to locate something that's rolled under your bed. It could be especially important if you feel low and want to test your blood glucose but the power is out.

854 **GOOF-PROOF YOUR HOME** ■ Do a safety check of your home for potential hazards: rugs that can slide and trip you, slippery bathtubs, highly waxed floors. All of this can cause leg or hip fractures.

Your local Visiting Nurse Service may offer occupational therapists who can help you with safety issues.

855 **KEEP A STASH OF EMERGENCY SUPPLIES** ■ Between blizzards and blackouts (and hurricanes, too), you must keep emergency supplies on hand, especially if you live alone.

Besides the extra drugs and equipment mentioned in Chapter 1, you should have extra lightbulbs, several flashlights, and lots of extra batteries, a couple of transistor radios (one may fade out after a week of continuous use), a first-aid kit, at least five gallons of water, and lots of candles with sturdy candle holders and matches.

Also a week's supply of canned food that you can eat cold in an emergency. My favorites are mostly 100 percent protein: chicken breast, salmon, and tuna, but I'd also include some canned ravioli in case I needed carbohydrates. *Make sure you have a hand-operated can opener so that you can get at this food during a power shortage!*

856 ***ANOTHER*** **ALARM SYSTEM?** ■ A number of companies sell medical alarm systems that can be very handy if you have a chronic disease. You wear an electronic pendant on a cord around your neck, and if you have an emergency, you press the button.

This activates a two-way system to call the monitoring center. You don't have to be able to reach your phone. Someone from the center will contact you immediately, twenty-four hours a day, and will then phone a designated friend or relative and the Emergency Medical Service, if necessary.

The cost seems to be pretty standard, with most of the companies charging approximately $30 a month.

857 POST MEDICAL EMERGENCY INFORMATION IN ALL THE RIGHT PLACES ■ Put this information on two sheets of paper on which you have drawn a big red border and title it "Medical Emergency Information." On each of them, write the same information: your name, medical problems, the drugs you are taking, any allergies or drug reactions, the name and phone number of your doctor, the name and phone number of your contact person, and your blood type, if you know it.

Stick one of the pages onto the inside of your front door with a magnet, and display the other prominently on your refrigerator door.

858 DON'T MISS A STEP ■ If your fuse box or circuit breakers are in your basement, paint the edge of every step with luminous white or Day-Glo paint. Then, if your lights go out, you'll manage to get safely down the basement stairs to change the fuse or reset the circuit breakers.

859 DON'T WAIT FOR PRINCE(SS) CHARMING ■ What are you waiting for? Living alone means never having to say, "Where's my bathrobe?" Waiting for somebody else to come along and give you a life is a double waste: You're missing weeks and years of private joys and adventures, and resenting some amorphous Providence for not delivering on your expectations. Making your own life as you go through it chapter by chapter is not only smarter and more efficient, taking responsibility for your attitudes and adventures puts you in charge.

9

Solving Special Problems

General

860 **HOW MUCH OF A WARNING DO YOU NEED?** ■ Many people got a warning recently, if they and their doctors were wise enough to heed it. "Prediabetes" refers to levels of blood glucose higher than normal, but less than the cutoff for a diagnosis of diabetes. Late in 2003, an international panel recommended new, lower guideline numbers defining prediabetes; the idea is to head the disease off at the pass before it's full-blown. If your fasting blood glucose reads between 100 and 125, or your nonfasting is 140 at any time of the day, head for the doctor now. Putting small changes into your lifestyle now could make the difference between developing diabetes or not.

861 **KEEP IT LEVEL** ■ Some people mistakenly imagine that type 2—insulin-resistant—diabetes is somehow less serious than type 1. Not so, and both require very close monitoring of blood-glucose levels. Type 2s have a very high risk of cardiovascular disease. Even if your doctor prescribes oral medication rather than insulin injections, both types of diabetes can lead to problems like kidney and eye problems and nerve damage. Keeping your blood-glucose level between 90 and 130 before meals, and less than 180 two hours after meals, is important no matter what diabetic medications you take.

862

WEB SITES FOR YOUR SPECIAL PROBLEMS ■ Try these organizations for more specific information. Many of them have an e-mail address, so that you can send them your questions directly.

American Foundation for Urologic Disease
1128 North Charles Street
Baltimore, MD 21201
(800) 242-2383 or (410) 468-1800
Web site: www.afud.org
E-mail: admin@afud.org

American Podiatric Medical Association
9312 Old Georgetown Road
Bethesda, MD 20814
(800) FOOTCARE or (301) 571-9200
Web site: www.apma.org
E-mail: askapma@apma.org

Centers for Disease Control and Prevention
National Center for Chromic Disease
Prevention and Health Promotion
Division of Diabetes Translation
Mail Stop K-10
4770 Buford Highway NE
Atlanta, GA 30341
(800) CDC-DIAB
Web site: www.cdc.gov/diabetes
E-mail: diabetes@cdc.gov

Juvenile Diabetes Research Foundation International
120 Wall Street
19th floor
New York, NY 10005
(800) 533-2873 or (212) 785-9500
Web site: www.jdrf.org
E-mail: info@jdrf.org

Lower Extremity Amputation Prevention Program
HRSA/BPH/DPSP
4350 East-West Highway
9th floor
Bethesda, MD 20814
(888) 275-4772
Web site: www.bphc.hrsa.gov/leap

National Diabetes Education Program
1 Diabetes Way
Bethesda, MD 20892-3600
(800) 438-5383
Web site: http://ndep.nih.gov

National Digestive Diseases Information Clearinghouse
2 Information Way
Bethesda, MD 20892
(800) 891-5389 or (301) 654-3810
Web site: www.niddk.nih.gov/health/digest/nddic.htm
E-mail: nddic@info.niddk.nih.gov

National Institute of Neurological Disorders and Stroke
PO Box 5801
Bethesda, MD 20824
(800) 891-5390 or (301) 654-4415
Web site: www.ninds.nih.gov

National Kidney and Urologic Diseases Information
3 Information Way
Bethesda, MD 20892-3580
(800) 891-5390 or (301) 654-4415
Web site: www.niddk.nih.gov/health/kidney/nkudic.htm

Pediatric Footwear Association
7150 Columbia Gateway Drive
Suite G
Columbia, MD 21046-1151
(800) 673-8447 or (410) 381-7278

863 **IT'S A CLOSED SYSTEM** ■ Realize that your body is a closed system: It's all connected. Your control of your diabetes—or the lack of it—will have a profound effect on your heart and blood vessels, your eyes, your kidneys, your feet, your nervous system—even your skin and your sex life.

864 **MINE THE INTERNET FOR SUPPORT AND INFORMATION** ■ The amount of responsible information on diabetes that is available on the Internet is truly amazing and heartening. Use google.com to refine your search and narrow it further by linking two or three key words instead of using just one.

I especially like the Web sites of the twenty-four medical boards that are members of the American Board of Medical Specialties (www.abms.org links to individual specialty boards) and the Insulin Dependent Diabetes Trust International (www.iddinternational.org) for a British and European perspective on diabetes.

865 **ARE YOU MARRIED TO A DIABETIC LIFESTYLE?** ■ The diabetes you prevent can be not only yours, but your significant other's. Studies done at the Royal London Hospital checked diabetes warning signals—weight, blood pressure, exercise habits, food choices, and smoking—and discovered that if one spouse already had diabetes, the other had significantly higher risk factors. Although diabetes isn't catching, a "diabetes lifestyle" can be. The researchers recommend getting screened if your partner has diabetes, and making walking dates together to share the time—*and* the benefits of regular exercise.

866 **DIABETES AIN'T DOOM, AND IT AIN'T DEPRESSION, EITHER** ■ Just like taking responsibility for managing your own blood-glucose levels, you can also manage your own happiness levels to a very large degree. Happiness researcher Dr. Sonja Lyubomirsky of the University of California, Riverside, says that about 40 percent of our happiness is influenced by what we deliberately do to make ourselves happy.

Her suggestions? Look for what's *right*—rather than what's wrong—with a day, a person, or a situation. Be grateful and kind as often as possible. Generate a rich and full social and friendship network. And make sure that you get enough rest, quiet, and solitude.

867 **PREVENTION BEATS TREATMENT** ■ As in all areas of life, prevention makes more sense than treatment. Prevention means intervening early to change and correct situations before they become problems. Prevention is much easier, faster, and cheaper. It's a much smarter move!

Pain Relief

868 **THE BRIGHT SIDE OF PAIN** ■ Amazingly, there *is* one. Pain is a symptom that something is not right and needs attention and care. When you can't feel pain immediately, as in various forms of neuropathy, you can suffer unknowingly, and your body might experience major damage.

That said, you'll find these resources useful:

869 THE PAIN FOUNDATION ■ For people in pain, the Pain Foundation offers information, advocacy, and support through online chat and discussion boards, publications, clinical trials, and finding help and information on complementary and alternative medicine. In addition to electronic and print newsletters, TPF offers the guides *Finding Help for Your Pain, The Pain Action Guide,* and a Pain Care Bill of Rights in English, Spanish, and Chinese. For more information, log on to www.painfoundation.org.

870 EVEN IF YOU HURT, YOU'RE NOT ALONE ■ The Pain Relief Network is an organization of pain patients, family members of people in pain, physicians, attorneys, and activists, all working toward achieving dignity and compassion for people who hurt. It's not only an online support group, it's also a political organizing group. With the mission statement of speaking for the 50 million people currently living in untreated disabling pain, PRN seeks to empower those people and demand that political leaders take notice and enable pain management to move forward legally in America. Log on to www.painreliefnetwork.org for more information.

871 RUB OUT YOUR PAIN? ■ Before taking more expensive and more invasive steps, see if an ancient Chinese therapy offers some pain relief. The book *Massage for Pain Relief; A Step-by-Step Guide* by Peijian Shen is an illustrated handbook. It offers techniques for safe, simple drug-free pain relief, using Chinese massage and pressure techniques to ease pain and prevent its return.

Hypoglycemia

872 DON'T LEAVE HOME WITHOUT IT ■ Keep glucose tablets or a roll of Lifesavers in your purse or briefcase, another stash in your desk, and still another under your pillow.

When your blood glucose drops like a rock, you want this help within easy reach.

873 **HAVE A SLIDING SCALE** ■ Discuss with your doctor if it's appropriate to have one plan if your blood glucose drops to around 55–60, another, more radical plan if it drops to 35–40—or whether "more of the same" is right for you.

874 **GLUCAGON: NOT IF YOU LIVE ALONE** ■ Glucagon is a wonderful first-response remedy for hypoglycemia, but it is useless if you live alone. If your blood glucose sinks so low that you need a glucose injection, you're not going to have the brain power or coordination to give yourself an injection, or to call a neighbor you've trained to do it.

875 **GLUCAGON'S SHORT SHELF LIFE** ■ Glucagon remains potent for only eighteen months. Check the expiration date when you pick up your glucagon kit at the pharmacy. Make a note in your daybook for December 31: "Glucagon expires (date) get a new one" and transfer it to the appropriate month of next year's daybook.

876 **IF YOU MUST CHOOSE** ■ It's far from the ideal solution, but if you must choose between high and low blood-glucose levels, you will damage your body much less by having a blood glucose over 200 than a blood glucose under 50 for one hour.

877 **FOR DRIVERS ONLY** ■ There are countless horror stories about people with diabetes causing car accidents because of a hypoglycemic attack. Probably about as many as about people suffering heart attacks at the wheel and crashing.

To be safe, test your blood glucose just before you pick up your car keys—even if it means testing three or four more times a day. And if you suddenly feel dizzy when you're at the wheel, pull off the road for a few minutes, get out of your car, and eat a few glucose tablets.

878 **CHECKING FOR HYPOGLYCEMIA? TEST HERE ONLY** ■ Most of the time, it's OK to use blood from your arm, thigh, or calf. But when you are checking for possible hypoglycemia, only finger sticks are accurate. It's not unusual to get a blood-glucose reading of 70 from your forearm, but only 40 from your finger.

879 **TIGHT CONTROL MAY INCREASE SEVERE HYPOGLYCEMIA** ■ Type 1 diabetics who are controlling their diabetes intensively are more likely to experience severe hypoglycemia than people with diabetes using ordinary control.

If this profile fits you and you experience hypoglycemia as often as once a week, ask your doctor to evaluate your drugs and dosages.

Sick Days

880 **SICK DAYS REQUIRE AT LEAST TWO PLANS** ■ Most books and magazines for people with diabetes urge us, "Have a plan for sick days." But I think we need at least two. We need one plan for fever and colds, but when we can eat normally, another when we can't keep any food down and have diarrhea.

Set up these plans now. When you're really sick, you're not thinking coherently enough to do it.

881 **AVOID DEHYDRATION** ■ Dehydration is a serious problem faced by people with diabetes when they get sick. Among the symptoms that increase the risk of dehydration are fever, vomiting, and diarrhea. Drink at least two quarts of water every day—more if you can stand it.

Ask your doctor whether you need to increase your salt intake to keep your electrolytes in balance, as you may have lost sodium as well as fluids.

882

SICK DAYS ARE LIKE HIGH-STRESS DAYS ■ Your body's response to sickness is very similar to its response to stress. Your blood-glucose level can rise 100–200 points overnight—and it's not because you overate.

Sick days just a fact of life—for some diabetics perhaps a little more frequent in our lives. But you have plans in place to deal with both high-stress days and sick days.

883

SICK DAYS MEAN MORE INSULIN ■ You will probably have to use more insulin when you are sick. Discuss with your doctor how many more units of insulin—and which types—for every 50 points of increased blood glucose. And check in with your doctor every day that you are sick; it may save a trip to the emergency room.

Thinking Clearly

884

"BRAIN FOG" AND HOW TO LIFT IT ■ Often "brain fog" is caused by high blood-glucose levels (over 200) for at least a week. High sugars actually thicken the blood. The farther from the heart and the smaller the blood vessel, the more slowly the blood will move and the less efficiently it will deliver oxygen and remove wastes from the tissues. The brain is so sensitive to being well nourished and cleaned of wastes that it is the most affected part of the body when sugars skyrocket.

If you can keep your sugars down to normal levels for at least a week, you will definitely notice the difference in your thinking!

885

MORE ABOUT MEMORY IMPAIRMENT ■ Check your carbohydrate intake before you think of impending

Alzheimer's. A recent study whose goal was to determine the impact of acute carbohydrate consumption on memory found that eating as little as 50 grams of quickly absorbed carbohydrate (½ bagel and white grape juice) produced significant memory deficits in people with type 2 diabetes.

Eyes

886 **LET 'EM CALL YOU "STAR," JUST WEAR YOUR SHADES** ■ Eye problems are much more prevalent among people who have had diabetes for a while. The quickest, easiest way to head off forming cataracts is to wear sunglasses in bright sunlight to forestall the lens of the eye becoming opaque and the retinas becoming less sensitive.

887 **BOOST THE TYPE WITH YOUR BROWSER** ■ Is the type on the Internet Web sites too small for you to read comfortably? Increase the print size with your browser settings. If you use Internet Explorer, click on "View" in the menu and then click on "Text Size" to choose a larger print.

888 **CHANGE THE CURSOR ARROW, TOO** ■ Maybe that little black arrow is *too* little to see easily. Change it to something larger, more brightly colored—maybe even a cartoon character. The Internet provides lots of free choices.

889 **GET BETTER NIGHT-DRIVING VISION** ■ Drivers who have diabetes often report difficulty with night vision. The reason: the dark makes your pupils dilate more, and the more peripheral light that enters your eyes, the more nearsighted you become. For a quick and simple solution, turn on the map light in your car. The extra (nondirect) illumination will make your pupils contract a bit. The result is slightly better vision and depth perception. But remember: This is a situational Band-Aid, not a fix: Get to your eye doctor for a checkup if the problem continues for three days.

890 **TURN DOWN THE NIGHTTIME GLARE** ■ The pain and danger of nighttime glare can be minimized with a trip to the drugstore. Dry eyes are more hurt by—and less effective in—glare. In fact, the drier your eyes, the worse the problem. So sterile eyedrops, or blinking, or thinking about the end of the movie *Lad: A Dog* can alleviate the situation by moistening your eyeballs. Contact-lens wearers, especially, should always carry eyedrops!

891 **NIGHT LIGHTS MAY PREVENT RETINOPATHY** ■ Researchers at Cardiff University in Wales have recently discovered that darkness causes hypoxia (oxygen deprivation) in the retinas of patients with type 2 diabetes. The scientists believe that the hypoxia may spur the tissue changes that occur in diabetic retinopathy. Light filtering through closed eyelids seems to prevent this oxygen starvation, so it may be wise to sleep with the light on.

Note: This was a very small study—only seven patients—so it lacks statistical significance. However, keeping the light near your bed on all night seems a very small, safe price to pay for preventing or delaying diabetic retinopathy.

892 **KEEP YOUR EDGE** ■ Impaired vision can cause major accidents when you are using sharp tools. To avoid bloodshed—yours—take an extra moment to ask yourself, "Where is my other hand? Where are all my fingers?"

893 **THE SHERLOCK HOLMES STRATEGY** ■ Keep at least one magnifying glass handy. Magnifying glasses come in a variety of strengths. Some combine two magnifications—like 2× and 5× in a single lens; some include battery-operated lights. Many have cords so that you can wear them around your neck. Magnifying glasses are a very inexpensive, low-tech solution to impaired-vision problems.

894 **THOSE MYSTERIOUS BLACK-AND-BLUE MARKS ARE IMPORTANT** ■ You start to get dressed in the morning or undressed at night—and there's a black-and-blue mark that you absolutely can't recall. These little mysteries shouldn't be ignored. Bumping into furniture can be the first symptom of impaired vision.

895 **DEALING WITH DIMINISHED VISION** ■ After "losing" a black plastic remote on a Black Watch plaid-sheeted bed for two days, which jacked up my stress level and my blood glucose, when I found it, I stuck strips of neon yellow adhesive tape on the remote. Now I can find it immediately.

896 **GAZE DEEPLY INTO YOUR EYES** ■ Does a full moon make you want to gaze deeply into a pair of eyes? Great—make that shiny orb your monthly reminder to spend an extra few minutes checking the reflections that indicate your cholesterol levels.

In front of the mirror, in good light, look at the skin around your eyes and eyelids. High blood-cholesterol levels often create visible signs, like fatty growth on the lids or around the eyes. Also, check around the irises of your eyes: Are there new gray fatty deposits around each iris?

Of course, this is no substitute for having your doctor do blood-chemistry tests, but it's one more way for you to assist in monitoring your own health.

897 **MAKE YOUR EYE DOCTOR YOUR SECOND-BEST FRIEND** ■ No more just getting glasses from an optician, or having the discount-superstore eye doc give you a prescription after you read the eye chart. People with diabetes are susceptible to several specific diabetic eye diseases, and regular checkups by a qualified specialist can screen for problems and literally save our sight. In addition to diabetic retinopathy, a leading cause of blindness, specialists will also screen for cataracts and glaucoma, which are twice as likely in diabetics as in the rest of the population.

Please get a dilated-eye exam at least twice a year, especially if you've been diabetic for several years.

898 **YOUR EYES AREN'T ONLY *YOUR* PROBLEM** ■ The National Eye Institute estimates that as many as 45 percent of all diagnosed diabetics have some degree of diabetic retinopathy, and as many as 4 million Americans suffer from the disease, with an estimated 25,000 people a year going blind from this disorder. It's one of the leading causes of blindness among working-age Americans, and costs the federal government almost $14,000 a year per person in Social Security benefits, lost income-tax revenues, and health-care expenditures. Screening and treatment to prevent vision loss could save the government more than $100 million a year—and preserve the eyesight of thousands of people. Uncle Sam wants you—to get your eyes checked!

899 **THOSE FUNNY LITTLE YELLOW SPOTS ARE SERIOUS** ■ During every eye examination, your doctor should examine your retinas for little yellow spots called "drusen." They are an early-warning sign of macular degeneration, a disease which is a leading cause of blindness.

If your doctor finds these spots, you *must* check your vision every day with a quick, simple test.

Cover one eye and look at something with straight lines, like a piece of graph paper. Now cover the other eye and repeat. If any of these lines appear wavy or you see a blank spot, call your doctor and get a referral to a retina specialist immediately.

900 SKIDPROOF YOUR HOME ■ Most falls are caused by poor vision. To prevent falling, get rid of scatter rugs or put skidproof tape on all the corners so they won't slip.

Clothing, papers, shoes, and other objects should be moved off the floor so you don't trip over them. Secure electrical and phone cords, too.

And skidproof your feet. Wear shoes and slippers that have nonslip soles; don't wear socks alone.

901 HEIGHTEN THE CONTRAST ■ To make seeing easier, use plates and dishes with contrasting colored rims and utensils with brightly colored handles.

Paint doorways or find a creative way—like an appliquéd border—to dramatize the edges. Put reflector tape on every edge you can think of, then ask a friend to double-check to see if there's anything else that needs special marking.

902 LIGHTEN UP ■ According to the Visiting Nurse Service of New York, older people need three times as much light as younger people. Many people with diabetes also need a lot more light. You may need to use stronger bulbs or add more lamps to increase your comfort, visibility, and sense of security.

903 LABEL YOUR DRUGS CLEARLY ■ Those tiny little vials with even tinier print can drive us nuts and create a risk if we can't read the labels.

Make a special label for each drug. Take a 3" × 5" index card and print on it all the necessary details so large that you can read them very easily. Then slip the index card and the drug vial into a plastic bag. Now reading all the details and taking the right medication at the right time will be easy.

904

IF YOU COULD DO ONLY ONE THING FOR YOUR EYES ■ One factor most influences the onset and progression of retinopathy, according to continuing analysis of the Diabetes Control and Complications Trial (DCCT), which ended ten years ago.

This crucial factor is sustained low glycosolated hemoglobin A1C numbers. Your focusing on getting these numbers down—and keeping them there—may prevent or delay diabetic retinopathy.

Cardiovascular

905

PAY ATTENTION TO HAIR LOSS ■ Diabetic nerve damage is often felt; diabetic peripheral vascular damage often isn't.

If you're losing the hair on the lower part of your legs, bring it to your doctor's attention quickly. Hair loss here can be a symptom of vascular disease, and curbing this complication can prevent amputation later.

906

CIGARETTES SHOULD BE YOUR OWN WORST ENEMY ■ People with diabetes need to do all they can to improve and maintain good circulation. Smoking destroys capillaries (your tiniest blood vessels) and circulation, especially in your hands and feet, which are at great risk, along with your kidneys and eyes. Stopping is the only smart move, and many medical groups have programs to help you. If you truly haven't been able to quit yet, then cut down as much as you can. (Doctors tell me that if you can limit your smoking to that one cigarette with your morning coffee—and wind up throwing away the package because the cigarettes are too stale, then you're probably not harming yourself.)

907

KNOW YOUR RISK ■ The National Institutes of Health warns that middle-aged people with type 2 diabetes have the same high risk of heart attack as people without diabetes who have already had one heart attack. Monitoring carbohydrates isn't usually enough to manage blood-glucose levels. It's also important to watch your saturated- and trans-fat intake because high cholesterol levels are also a complication of diabetes.

908 **PESSIMISM IS MORE THAN AN ATTITUDE** ■ Research has shown that pessimism can increase the number of T-suppressor cells. In addition to interfering with your immune system, these cells can raise the risk of developing heart disease. Believing that your health problems are not controllable or treatable is a dangerous supposition: It even affects the intensity of your pursuing treatment.

909 **HEART DISEASE IS NOT A MALE PROBLEM** ■ Although heart disease tends to be classified and treated as a "male" disease by the medical community, it is the single greatest health risk for women today—greater than stroke and all cancers combined. More American women die of heart disease each year than of the next seven causes of death combined. Heart disease actually kills more women than men, although typically it strikes ten years later.

Make sure that you discuss reducing cardiovascular risk with your doctor. Prevention is crucial because most women who die suddenly of a heart attack had no history of cardiovascular disease, but did have at least one risk factor: high cholesterol, diabetes, hypertension, obesity, or smoking.

910 **GET THE RIGHT TESTS** ■ For women, a treadmill stress test is less accurate and predictive than it is for men. For proper diagnosis and treatment, it should be combined with an echocardiogram or a nuclear-imaging test.

911

ATRIAL FIBRILLATION CAN BE MORE SERIOUS IN WOMEN ■ Atrial fibrillation (AF), an abnormally fast and irregular heartbeat, is the most common form of cardiac arrhythmia. Although men are more likely than women to develop AF, women have twice the risk of stroke after developing it, according to the landmark Framingham heart study reported in August 2003.

Atrial fibrillation doesn't always show up in EKGs because those tests are so brief—only about ten seconds. If your symptoms persist, you may need a longer test with a portable heart monitor.

As a diabetic, you are already at risk for atrial fibrillation and other arrhythmias. Quitting smoking is the smartest thing you can do to reduce your risk because smoking triples the risk of arrhythmias.

912

GENDER DIFFERENCES IN SYMPTOMS OF HEART ATTACK AND STROKE ■ You probably know the traditional symptoms of heart attack and stroke in men; they've been dramatized often enough. The most common male symptom of heart attack is a sharp, clutching pain in the chest that often radiates down the arm. The most common male symptoms of stroke are a sudden weakness, numbness, or lack of coordination on one side of the body, or sudden inability to speak.

In women, the signs are much more subtle and diffuse, which makes diagnosis and immediate treatment much more difficult. Heart-attack symptoms include unexplained headaches, nausea, breathlessness, and palpitations. Stroke symptoms include pain, headache, changes in consciousness, and disorientation. Perhaps Nieca Goldberg, M.D., founder and chief of the Women's Health Program at New York's Lenox Hill Hospital, summed it up best in the title of her book: *Women Are Not Small Men.*

Neuropathy

913
QUALITATIVE SENSORY TESTING: BIG NAME, LITTLE TESTS ■ Don't be concerned if your doctor recommends "qualitative sensory testing." It sounds imposing, but it's actually the use of pressure, vibration, temperature, and other stimuli to check for possible nerve damage. QST is used to identify and quantify sensation loss and excessive nerve irritability. The test can help your doctor plan specific treatment.

914
WEAK LEGS? CHECK FOR PROXIMAL NEUROPATHY ■ People with type 2 diabetes and older people may experience weakness in their legs or difficulty standing after they've been sitting for a long time. The cause may be proximal neuropathy: nerve damage also known as "femoral neuropathy" or "lumbosacral plexus neuropathy." The condition starts with pain in either of the thighs, hips, buttocks, or legs, usually on one side of the body. It's worth bringing to your doctor's attention; treatment for the weakness or pain is usually needed.

915
IF YOU'RE THE ONLY ONE SWEATING, IT'S NOT JUST HOT IN HERE ■ Diabetic nerve damage can affect the nerves that control sweating. When autonomic neuropathy keeps your sweat glands from working properly, your body loses the ability to regulate your temperature. Nerve damage can also cause profuse perspiring at night, or while you're eating. Women of a certain age who have diabetes should bring unusual sweating problems to their doctor's attention—it might not be hot flashes.

Joints and Muscles

916 **MUSCLE CRAMPS CAN MEAN MORE THAN OVEREXERTION** ■ If you're getting leg or other muscle cramps, give a thought to the possible causes. Your cramps could be the results of overexertion, but they can also signal dehydration or electrolyte imbalances. If clenched leg muscles recur without obvious triggers, check with your physician.

917 **ELECTROMYOGRAPHY: THE TEST THAT SOUNDS WORSE THAN IT IS** ■ People with diabetes can experience decreased muscle responses, and doctors may want to test how well muscles respond to the electrical signals transmitted by nearby nerves. The idea of running electrical pulses into your muscles sounds scary, but it's neither as fearsome nor as painful as it sounds. Electromyograhy (EMG) displays your muscles' electrical activity on a screen and isolates the slower or weaker responses that suggest damage. This test can also be done at the same time as nerve-conduction studies and, for most people, is not particularly irritating or painful.

918 **THE PSI FACTOR** ■ This psi has nothing to do with ESP. It stands for pounds per square inch, a measurement of stress used by mechanical engineers and architects.

Here's why it applies to you. If you are seriously overweight, you are putting your knees and ankles at very great risk, damaging them with every step you take. There is a simple mathematical formula to estimate the pounds per square inch pressure on your knees and ankles. It is only an estimate because it ignores your height, and the taller you are, the more stress you are putting on your knees and ankles. However, it also underestimates the psi impact because the formula treats the entire area of the joint as it were all bone—not flesh and bone—and your bone really bears your weight.

The formula for calculating the pounds per square inch on each joint is simple:

Measure your knee (or ankle) with a tape measure. This is the circumference.

Divide by 3.14 (pi) to get your joint's diameter.

Divide by 2 to get your joint's radius.

Then multiply the radius by itself and then by 3.14.

Yes, this is your old high school geometry formula for calculating the area of a circle. It really doesn't matter that your joint is shaped irregularly, and is not a pure circle. The circumference controls the area; try experimenting with a string and you'll see.

To bring the damage home, let's plug in some numbers:

If your knee measures 20" in circumference, its diameter is 6.37" and its radius is 3.18". Its area is 31.8 square inches. If you weigh 150 pounds, the pressure on your knee is 4.7 psi. (A square inch is an area about the size of the first joint of your thumb.) If you weigh 300 pounds, the pressure is 9.4 psi.

Your ankle's circumference is generally about 60 percent the size of your knee's, so the psi numbers are almost twice as large.

Is it any wonder that seriously overweight people are at substantial risk for osteoarthritis and other joint and muscle problems?

Will knowing the potential damage persuade you to lose some weight? I hope so!

919 **STEP UP** ■ Does one knee hurt more than the other? This trick may lessen your pain: When you step up on a curb or climb steps, lead off with your "good" leg. When you step down from the curb or go downstairs, start with your "bad" leg.

920 **DEALING WITH FROZEN SHOULDER** ■ "Frozen shoulder" covers all causes of motion loss in the shoulder joint. Like many joint problems, it affects women more than men, approximately 10 to 20 percent of people with diabetes, and usually begins between the ages of forty and sixty-five.

According to the American Academy of Orthopaedic Surgeons, frozen shoulder is probably caused by underlying inflammation that makes the capsule surrounding the shoulder joint thicken and contract, so that the upper arm bone (humerus) has less room to move around.

Nonsurgical treatment, which should be tried first, includes anti-inflammatory drugs and muscle relaxants, heat or ice therapies, physical therapy combined with stretching exercises done at home to help restore motion and function, and corticosteroid injections.

Arthroscopic surgery is used if there is no improvement after several months. It must be followed by an exercise program to restore function and maintain the range of motion.

921

TANDEM POINT^{SM} THERAPY MAY HELP ■ Tandem Point^{SM} therapy can relieve pain and/or loss of motion that may be caused by muscle contraction. This form of physical therapy is a combination of acupressure and massage that involves applying pressure simultaneously to a trigger point and one or more other points, then stretching through the trigger point.

Tandem Point^{SM} therapy is fast; according to a presentation made at the National Institutes of Health, improvement is usually seen after one visit.

Gastrointestanal Tract

922

TO OUTWIT GASTROPARESIS, TRY SPACING YOUR MEALS ■ Neuropathy from extended high blood-glucose levels—diabetic gastroparesis—can take its toll on stomach nerves, causing nausea, indigestion, belching, and vomiting. Doctors suggest battling the milder symptoms of stomach-nerve damage by eating small, frequent meals, avoiding fats, and eating less fiber. For more severe symptoms, doctors may prescribe erythromycin to speed digestion, metoclopramide to speed digestion and help relieve nausea, or other drugs that can affect stomach-enzyme secretions.

923 **SLOW GASTRIC EMPTYING DELAYS EVERYTHING** ■ It usually takes about two hours for food and drink to move out of your stomach and on to your small intestine. In slow gastric emptying, it takes at least four or five hours. Slow gastric emptying delays the absorption of drugs as well as food. Pills sit in the stomach rather than passing through quickly. This alters the action of oral hypoglycemics.

Nausea and heartburn after eating are two major symptoms of slow gastric emptying. If you experience them frequently, you should probably see a gastroenterologist.

924 **BALANCING ACT** ■ If your blood-glucose levels run high and low and seem frequently to be 180 degrees out of sync, the problem may be that your stomach is emptying more slowly. Speak to your doctor about adjusting your insulin medication and possibly your oral hypoglycemics so that it matches your digestion time better.

925 **THE LINK BETWEEN DIABETES AND CHRONIC DIARRHEA** ■ Like many other systems of the body, your gastrointestinal system is affected by diabetes. Because intestinal movement can be slowed down (gastroparesis), which is usually caused by neuropathy of the autonomic nervous system, there is a population explosion of the bacteria that normally live in the intestine. Drugs that stimulate the muscular action of the intestines and antibiotics like erythromycin will usually cure chronic diarrhea.

Kidneys

926 **WATCH YOUR ALBUMIN AND CREATININE** ■ Guidelines from the National Kidney Foundation suggest that people with diabetes, hypertension, or a family history of kid-

ney disease should get a urine test for albumin and a blood test for creatinine. The albumin test indicates impaired function (a qualitative
test), and the creatinine test tells your doctor how efficiently your kidneys are functioning (a quantitative test).

927 KNOW YOUR NUMBERS I: ALBUMIN ■ Your doctor
should be having your urine tested for protein regularly. When your kidneys are functioning normally, they filter out a
protein called albumin from the urine. (Tiny amounts of albumin are
called "microalbumin.") As kidney function declines, more and more
albumin escapes into the urine.

Get a copy of every lab test and examine it. According to Quest
Diagnostics, numbers between 0 and 30 are normal. Ask your doctor
to evaluate any higher number that might be abnormal.

928 KNOW YOUR NUMBERS II: CREATININE ■ Creatinine
is a white crystalline compound that is a component
of urine. Results are converted to mg./liter. Not only should you look
at whether the results of any one test are normal, but you and your
doctor should compare them to the past two or three results to make
sure that they are not sliding slowly from normal to abnormal.

929 KNOW YOUR NUMBERS III: GLOMERULAR FILTRATION
RATE (GFR) ■ Simply put, the glomerular filtration
rate (GFR) tells you and your doctor at what percentage your kidneys
are doing their work. The National Kidney Foundation lists six stages
of chronic kidney disease, based on your GFR:

STAGE	DESCRIPTION	GLOMERULAR FILTRATION RATE (GFR)
At increased risk	*Risk factors* for kidney disease (e.g., diabetes, high blood pressure, family history, older age, ethnic group)	More than 90

STAGE	DESCRIPTION	GLOMERULAR FILTRATION RATE (GFR)
1	Kidney damage (protein in the urine) and *normal* GFR	More than 90
2	Kidney damage and *mild* decrease in GFR	60 to 89
3	*Moderate* decrease in GFR	30 to 59
4	*Severe* decrease in GFR	15 to 29
5	*Kidney failure* (dialysis or kidney transplant needed)	Less than 15

930 EARLY KIDNEY DISEASE IN TYPE 1 DIABETICS MAY BE REVERSIBLE ■ Microalbuminuria (small amounts of protein in the urine), an early sign of kidney disease, might be reversed with early detection and good diabetes control, according to researchers at the Joslin Diabetes Center, who reported the results of their study in the June 5, 2003, issue of the *New England Journal of Medicine.*

Bruce Perkins, M.D., M.P.H., F.R.C.P., the lead author of the six-year study, reported: "In this early stage, we found kidney injury is still a dynamic process that can either get worse or get better—even revert back to normal."

Factors that made a difference in returning to normal kidney function included early detection of microalbuminuria, a glycosolated hemoglobin A1C of less than 8.0, systolic blood pressure less than 115, total cholesterol less than 198, and fasting triglycerides under 145.

It's wonderful to have this good news!

Feet

931 WHY ARE ALL THESE TIPS NECESSARY? ■ This section of "Solving Special Problems" contains more tips than any other because foot problems can develop so quickly and are so dangerous. Where cardiovascular and other problems may develop

slowly, over years, foot problems are the major cause of diabetics' trips to the emergency room.

932 DON'T BE DE-FEET-ED ■ Until I interviewed a doctor with years of experience in family medicine, I was under the misapprehension that most diabetic patients' trips to the emergency room were for hypoglycemia.

Not so. Many more visits are for foot problems, which often start small, but become worse very rapidly. Taking the best care of your feet will keep you out of emergency rooms and hospitals.

933 YOUR ODDS ARE ONE IN FOUR, SO START WATCHING NOW ■ Without vigilance and prevention, your odds are one in four. Of the 16 million Americans with diabetes, 4 million will develop foot problems related to the disease. Poor circulation can cause a lack of sensitivity of loss of the ability to feel pain, heat, and cold. That makes it possible to develop cuts, scrapes, blisters, or pressure sores without feeling them. And if minor injuries go untreated, complications could lead to ulceration and possibly even amputation. So if you "just don't bother" to check your feet every day, remember your one-in-four odds.

934 HAVING COLD FEET MEANS MORE THAN RELUCTANCE ■ At the very least, cold feet are a sign of poor peripheral (your hands and feet) circulation. More seriously, cold feet might be a symptom of neuropathy. Keep your feet warm with the most comfortable socks you can find—cashmere-blend knee socks go on sale the day after Christmas.

Tell your doctor about your cold feet at your next appointment.

935 NEVER USE AN ELECTRIC BLANKET ON YOUR FEET ■ If you have neuropathy, you could burn your feet with an electric blanket and not realize the damage until it's too late. You can use the electric blanket on the rest of your body, and a hot-water bottle is safe for your feet. (Or teach your cats or dogs to sleep on your feet—that's the origin of Three-Dog Night.)

936 CUSTOM ORTHOTICS MAY NOT BE NECESSARY ■ Try the orthotics and insoles sold at your pharmacy first. In one recent visit, I found over twenty different types, none of which cost more than $15 for the largest men's size. Definitely worth trying!

937 FOOT NEUROPATHY? INCREASE YOUR FLEXIBILITY AND CIRCULATION ■ When your toes get stiff and inflexible, walking becomes difficult. You may even need to use a walker.

Try this little trick to increase your circulation and flexibility. Pick up marbles in your toes. Start with large marbles and graduate to small ones. You can also pick up napkin rings with your toes and put them on a spike. (There are many toys for infants and toddlers consisting of concentric rings that are placed on a peg. Look for these at yard sales.)

938 FOOT ULCERS ARE DEADLY ■ True story: Several months ago, I ran into a neighborhood friend and we brought each other up to date. She knows I have diabetes—but not that I was writing this book—and told me that one of her neighbors, a woman in her forties with poorly controlled diabetes, had been found dead in her apartment several days earlier. The cause of death was an untreated foot ulcer.

Without belaboring the point, untreated foot ulcers can kill you. If you have a sore on your foot, call your doctor *immediately.*

939 "DIABETIC FOOT" COVERS A LOT OF GROUND ■ "Diabetic foot" sums up a cluster of serious problems common to people with diabetes: primarily, neuropathy, vasculopathy (circulatory problems), infections, and poor wound healing.

If your doctor diagnoses your problem as "diabetic foot," ask for a more specific diagnosis and a detailed treatment plan.

940 "CHARCOT FOOT" MEANS ONLY ONE THING ■ Charcot foot is a specific disease. It begins with neuropathy and progresses quickly to a degenerative arthritis in which the ligaments and joint surfaces of the metatarsal and tarsal bones disintegrate.

According to the American Diabetes Association, 60 to 70 percent of people with diabetes develop peripheral neuropathy that can lead to Charcot foot, whose onset usually occurs in middle-aged patients who have diabetes for fifteen to twenty years. Of course, poorly controlled blood glucose makes the situation worse—and earlier.

Treatment can be complex and can take months. The damaged joint must be stabilized for at least two months, which means that it must not bear any weight. Patients are prescribed bed rest and/or a walking cast and crutches. If there is no improvement, surgery may be necessary.

941 CHECK YOUR FEET MORNING OR NIGHT ■ Your feet need checking daily. So mentally tie foot-checking to something else you do without fail, like brushing your teeth or locking the door. Once you've linked this task into a routine, it will take as little conscious effort to remember checking your feet as it does to brush your teeth.

942 SOCKS MIGHT BE YOUR BEST FRIEND ■ Anything that rubs or abrades your feet is very bad. Anything that protects and soothes them is very good. So start your collection of colorful, fine-combed cotton socks. The importance of the warmth, protection, and absorbency of soft cotton socks can't be overemphasized.

943 HURTING? YOUR DRUGSTORE HAS TOPICAL HELP ■ People with diabetes often experience pain in their feet as the nerves become damaged from continued high blood-glucose levels. Some people report lying awake at night, trying to sleep despite their discomfort. Go for a topical analgesic: "Stop Pain" spray or even Anbesol—a product made for teething babies and oral cold-sore sufferers—can help. If it's safe enough to put in your mouth, it's safe enough for unbroken skin on your foot. By dulling or removing the pain temporarily, you are freed to think about something else, or even get a good night's sleep.

944 **DIABETIC SOCKS ARE NOT A CROCK** ■ Don't make the mistake of thinking that all products pitched to people with diabetes are after your money. So-called "diabetic socks" can change your life! Some are made with wider tops because tight or binding socks can restrict your circulation, which is the last thing you want or need. Some are made with patented "miracle fibers" that wick away moisture and/or prevent rubbing and chafing. If your feet are giving you any trouble at all, check out socks designed to answer these problems. Yes, you'll pay more for them; and yes, anything that helps your feet last throughout your lifetime is worth that extra outlay.

945 **WHY GO BAREFOOT WHEN SLIPPERS WERE MADE JUST FOR YOU?** ■ The selection and ingenuity behind foot-problem slippers will amaze you. The less-love term is "edema footwear, also known as diabetic footwear," but the comfort and relief available from these specialty products will surprise you when you check them out. Special shoes and slippers have been designed to help those suffering from edema (swelling), diabetes, sensitive skin, misshapen feet, and other problems. And they're not your grandmother's black old-lady shoes. Attractive and comfortable styles now exist in extra-wide, no-inside-seams, down-lined—whatever you need to prevent or relieve problems. Don't wait until foot pain sends you looking for them—wearing them preventively is doubly smart.

946 **ASK YOUR DOCTOR ABOUT PLASTAZOTE** ■ Footwear and orthotics play a key role in foot care for people

with diabetes, both to prevent and to help heal. Plastazote foam is the most often used material for protecting diabetic feet that have lost their sensitivity, and orthotics utilizing it can relieve pressure "hot spots" by conforming to heat and pressure. Because Plastazote shapes to your feet, it provides both comfort and protection. Ask your doctor about shoe inserts made with this product, or a similar one.

947 **WATCH YOUR FEET IN WINTER** ■ One of the hardest things for some people to remember is that "familiar" does not equal "safe." Just because you've lived in Buffalo or Cleveland for years and are used to the weather, that doesn't mean your feet won't need special attention in the winter. Cold feet—especially wet cold feet—can be disastrous for people with diabetes. Seamless socks and lined waterproof boots are vital in the winter! Check your feet often; someone without diabetic neuropathy might feel developing frostbite, but you might not. Keep your feet warm and dry. If possible, have someone else dig your car out of the snowbank or shovel the walk. And carry an extra pair of shoes and socks with you or in your car, in case yours become wet.

948 **BEACH SHOES ARE A MUST** ■ Walking barefoot in the sand really works only in the movies. The sand that looks so inviting from a distance is actually mined liberally with sharp-edged shells and discarded can pull-tabs. And it's *hot!* Always wear shoes at the beach or on hot pavement, and put sunscreen on the tops of your feet. Semirigid soled, net-topped beach shoes make you look like a savvy veteran surfer—too smart to risk unnecessary hazards as you enjoy nature at the shore.

949 **GO WITH THE FLOW** ■ One of the smartest, effortless things you can do for your feet is to keep the blood flow going. Put your feet up when you are sitting, and don't cross your legs for long periods. No tight socks, elastic, or garters on your legs. And if you've been sitting awhile, wiggle your toes and rotate your ankles to improve blood flow in your feet and legs.

950 THE RIGHT WAY TO TREAT YOUR FEET ■ Soothing emollients on your feet are always welcomed, but rub skin lotion or cream *only* on the tops and bottoms of your feet. Don't put lotion between your toes; the warm, moist climate there could invite athlete's foot and other nasties. And note any changes on your feet that last too long.

How long is too long? Call your doctor immediately if a cut, sore, blister, or bruise on your foot does not clearly begin to heal after one day.

951 BREAK NEW SHOES IN SLOWLY ■ Never wear new shoes all day away from home; carry a spare pair with you just in case. Break new shoes in first at home. If they are uncomfortable, return them. You do not want to risk getting a blister because blisters can become infected and turn dangerous in a matter of hours.

952 ANODYNE THERAPY: WORTH CHECKING OUT ■ If foot ulcers or damaged nerves in your legs and feet give you grief, consider anodyne therapy. In this treatment, near-infrared light-emitting "paddles" are placed over damaged areas to reduce pain by improving your circulation. You'll need twelve sessions of forty minutes each, according to podiatrists, but results are reported to last for one year, with 95 percent of patients obtaining relief. For more information, call (800) 521-6664, or log on to www.anodynetherapy.com.

953 CASTING CALL ■ Untreated foot sores or ulcers may lead to amputation. Previously, these problems were treated with special shoes, but many patients were "noncompliant": they took the shoes off.

To solve this problem, researchers at the Pitié Salpêtrière teaching hospital in Paris invented a virtually irremovable fiberglass cast that helps diabetic foot sores heal faster than the shoes did. That's probably because only one determined person in the study was able to remove the cast, compared with many who stopped wearing the shoes.

954 **KEEP YOUR FEET DRY WHEN GARDENING** ■ Heavy watering means taking special care of your feet. Apply petroleum jelly or a urea-based lotion on the bottoms of your feet, and then cover with cotton socks and rubber boots. Not only will your feet feel completely dry, but your feet will think they're getting a spa treatment.

955 **HAVE YOUR FAVORITE SHOES STOPPED FITTING?** ■ If your favorite shoes have stopped being comfy, it may be an early sign of foot trouble. Double-check by trying on several pairs of your favorites, especially at the beginning of spring and fall. Tightness can indicate swelling or "hot spots"—blisters waiting to happen. *Tell your doctor.*

956 **KEEP SOAKING TIME SHORT** ■ You'd think that soaking your feet for a while would alleviate dryness problems, but prolonged soaking actually *causes* dryness. Limit soaking your feet to ten minutes at a time, and dry them carefully, especially between your toes.

957 **BABY YOUR FEET WITH POWDER** ■ In order to prevent dampness between your toes, which can cause fungus to develop, keep the skin between your toes dry by using cotton swabs or powder. Baby powder has a pleasant unisex aroma, but many people find lavender more appealing, and women may prefer rose-scented powder.

958 **NAIL IT DOWN** ■ Thick or yellow toenails can be a symptom of two different diseases: one caused by a fungus, one by bacteria. Call your doctor as soon as you notice this problem. Like many others, treatment is easier and faster if the problem is caught early.

959 MIRROR, MIRROR ■ If you can't see your feet to examine them—tops *and soles*—use a mirror and a magnifying glass in a well-lighted area.

960 LEAVE CORNS AND CALLUSES TO YOUR DOCTOR ■ Having diabetes means that you shouldn't practice self-taught surgery on your feet. Do not cut corns or calluses; broken skin can lead to infection. However, you can use a pumice stone to smooth them. Rub gently *in one direction only* to avoid tearing the skin.

961 PEDICURE POINTERS ■ Spring and summer, a cruise, or a sunny resort are all invitations to show off our pretty feet. And that means a pedicure.

To prevent damage, you'll have to lay down the law to make sure the pedicurist doesn't do anything that could cause an infection. That means no cutting or shaving of cuticles or corns. Emery boards and pumice stones are safe.

Note: I urge people with diabetes to have their podiatrist trim their toenails rather than the pedicurist.

962 PUMP IT UP ■ A new device designed for home use increases circulation and lowers the risk of amputation. Peripheral arterial disease (PAD) is the culprit, and people with diabetes are especially susceptible because diabetes raises both cholesterol and triglyceride levels. Both are PAD risk factors.

This device—the ArtAssist—fits around the calf and foot, applying massagelike pressure. Says Ed Arkans, president and founder of ACI Medical, the manufacturer of ArtAssist, "Rapid, high-speed compression increases blood flow to the lower leg and to the skin in the foot." A small clinical study of men in their seventies at the State University of New York in Stony Brook found that the ArtAssist prevented amputations in 77 percent of the subjects.

963 SHOE SMARTS ■ Buy shoes that are long enough, wide enough, and deep enough so that they don't pinch, rub, or squeeze your feet. All of these irritations can cause blisters. Shop for shoes at the end of the day, when your feet are at their largest. And try them with the socks, stockings, or tights you plan to wear with them. You'll be able to gauge whether they fit properly, and you'll get a better idea of how they'll look together.

964 THE SYNERGY OF SOCKS ■ If your feet ache from cold or neuropathy, try putting on a second pair of soft, cushiony, nonbinding socks on top of the first pair. For reasons understood only by physicians, physicists, physiologists, and leprechauns, the effect is more than twice as soothing and warming as a single pair. Try it!

965 LENGTHENING YOUR ACHILLES TENDON MAY PREVENT THE RECURRENCE OF FOOT ULCERS ■ Diabetic foot ulcers can be healed and their recurrence can be prevented, according to a two-year study at the Washington University School of Medicine in St. Louis. All the participants received total-contact casts; half of them also had their Achilles tendon lengthened, outpatient surgery that generally takes only fifteen minutes. Two years after treatment, foot ulcers had recurred in 81 percent of the cast-only group, but in only 38 percent of the subjects who had undergone the Achilles tendon surgery.

Hands

966 BABY YOUR HANDS ■ Don't ignore your hands. Your feet bear the weight, so they are subject to more mechanical stress, but your hands have more nerves, muscles, and blood vessels, and are used more in more specialized ways. That means more problems can arise.

We diabetics and our doctors focus on our feet because foot problems are much more serious. But people with diabetes have many hand problems, too. They tend to be less serious and less exclusively diabetic, but they should not be ignored.

967

EASIER KITCHEN TOOLS ■ Little things can make a big difference in your quality of life. Gadgets that are easier to manipulate can diminish the pain in your hands and fingers considerably. Some of the most useful I've found are a ridged rubber mat about the size of a pot holder that makes it easier to open screw-top jars, and a can opener with ergonomic handles.

968

NON-CHILD-RESISTANT PRESCRIPTION BOTTLES MINIMIZE HAND PAIN ■ Child-resistant prescription bottles are hard to open, especially if you have arthritis or other hand problems. If you don't have small children, get your prescriptions in easy-to-open pop-top containers.

969

GLOVES AREN'T FOR WIMPS ■ Gloves protect your hands from chapping and dryness caused by cold and windburn. People with diabetes need to be especially protective of their hands to prevent skin damage and even possible frostbite. Try wearing knitted silk gloves under your winter gloves—they're available through outdoor and ski shops and catalogs—or wear two pairs of gloves at one time.

970

AMERICAN HOT WAX ■ A paraffin treatment for your hands can reduce arthritis pain and increase the flexibility of your hands and fingers. No need to visit a nail spa, unless you want to try a treatment first. You should be able to buy the whole kit to treat both hands and feet for under $60, and you can reuse the paraffin and use the treatment several times a week.

971 **CARPAL TUNNEL SYNDROME I: KNOW THE SYMPTOMS** ■ Your fingers may feel numb, or like pins and needles. If these strange feelings persist for more than a day—and especially if you spend a good part of the day at the computer or doing repetitive actions with your hands—carpal tunnel syndrome is a likely diagnosis.

972 **CARPAL TUNNEL SYNDROME II: IT'S ALL IN THE WRIST** ■ Carpal tunnel syndrome is caused by repeated physical stress to a small part of the wrist, which then squeezes a major nerve. High blood glucose may also alter collagen in your wrist, which can also increase pressure on this nerve.

973 **CARPAL TUNNEL SYNDROME III: SPLINT, STEROIDS, SURGERY** ■ The most conservative and sensible treatment starts with your doctor's splinting your wrist to keep it stabilized and free of pressure. You'll have to wear the splint as much as possible—even at night.

The next step is steroid injections to reduce the swelling putting pressure on the nerve. (Blood-glucose levels can shoot up for twenty-four hours after steroid injections.)

Surgery may work if your pain becomes severe, or if your hand and wrist muscles start to weaken noticeably.

974 **TRIGGER FINGER, TRIGGER THUMB** ■ They sound like fightin' words from a John Wayne western, but they're a common problem for people with diabetes over the age of forty.

Trigger finger and trigger thumb occur when the finger's flexor tendon or sheath thicken or swell, preventing normal, smooth gliding. When the tendon swells too much, it gets stuck and locks or clicks.

Your doctor can diagnose trigger finger and trigger thumb by examining your fingers and manipulating them, checking if there is a catching or locking as they move. X rays are not necessary.

Treatment is similar to that for carpal tunnel syndrome: splinting, sometimes taking aspirin or ibuprofen to reduce the swelling, and a steroid injection or surgery if necessary.

Teeth

975 **SIX-MONTH CHECKUPS ARE ESPECIALLY IMPORTANT** ■ People with diabetes are at high risk for tooth decay, periodontal (gum) disease, fungal infections of the mouth, and infection and delayed healing. Regular visits to your dentist can prevent these problems, or stop them in their earliest stages. Think of the difference between having a cavity filled and needing to have that tooth extracted and replaced!

976 **GET SCREENED FOR ORAL CANCER** ■ Make sure that your dentist examines your mouth for oral cancer once a year. Oral cancer is more prevalent in African-Americans, men, people over the age of forty-five, and people who use alcohol and tobacco (including smokeless types). However, there is no clear statistical correlation between people with diabetes and oral cancer.

Your dentist should examine the floor of your mouth, the front and sides of your tongue, and your soft palate to do a complete screening.

977 **MORE FREQUENT CLEANING SAVES BIG BUCKS** ■ Getting your teeth cleaned three or four times a year rather than twice can be a smart move. People with diabetes are more likely to develop plaque and tartar, which lead to gingivitis and periodontal disease, so more frequent professional cleaning can get rid of the plaque and tartar before they cause damage.

978 THIS THRUSH IS NO BIRD ■ If your blood-glucose levels are consistently too high, you may develop thrush, a fungus disease of the mouth characterized by white patches.

Thrush is not very serious, but it needs to be treated with oral antifungal medication, and it can raise your blood glucose substantially until it is cured.

If you develop thrush every few months, regard it as a sign that your immune system may need help. Keeping tighter control of your blood glucose is a key step.

979 ATTACK YOUR PLAQUE ■ Plaque is the sticky film on teeth that is produced by and encourages the growth of bacteria in your mouth. It is the first stage of periodontal disease and leads to the formation of calculus (calcified plaque), which builds up under the gums, forming pockets of infection.

Get rid of plaque by brushing and flossing at least twice a day, and you can avoid this nasty, expensive progression.

980 THE SUGAR IN YOUR SALIVA ■ You knew this was the culprit, didn't you? People with good glycemic control have no more periodontal disease than nondiabetics. But many types of bacteria thrive on sugars, and a warm, dark, high-sugar environment—like your mouth—is ideal for growing the germs that cause gum disease.

The better your blood-glucose control, the more you will protect your mouth from periodontal disease.

981 ANTIBIOTICS REDUCE RISK AFTER ORAL SURGERY ■ People with diabetes are at risk of infection anytime their skin is cut, and that includes oral surgery—especially because the human mouth is always teeming with bacteria.

Make it a habit to ask your dentist for antibiotics whenever you have even the most minor gum surgery. It can prevent major problems from arising.

Skin

982 **SAVE YOUR SKIN** ■ One of the side effects of diabetes is aged-looking skin as connective tissue breaks down. One home remedy to help you hold the line—or hold off the lines!—is jojoba butter mixed with the herb gotu kola. Studies have shown that gotu kola can strengthen collagen, and it's often used to treat burn victims. A trip to the health-food store for standardized extract of gotu kola containing 40 percent asiaticosides (the active ingredient) and jojoba butter will help make your skin look better.

983 **MINIMIZE DAMAGE FROM INSECT BITES** ■ The summer of 2003 brought a population explosion of biting insects to a large part of the United States. Many people with diabetes who hadn't been bitten in many years suddenly became human pincushions and blood banks. It's probably our sweeter blood that makes us such appealing targets.

Every one of these bites can become infected, and that's the problem. Prevent infection by washing the bites immediately with soap and water, putting triple antibiotic ointment (bacitracin + neomycin + polymyxin B) on them, and then covering them with small adhesive bandages.

984 **MINOR SKIN PROBLEMS IN GENERAL** ■ Except for "diabetic foot," **(Tip No. 939)**, most diabetic skin problems are minor, according to a New York dermatologist with over thirty years of experience. They deserve discussion because your knowing what they are and that they are not serious should alleviate your stress. Learn to recognize them and point them out to your doctor, but don't worry about them unless you notice a change in their appearance.

985 **MINOR SKIN PROBLEMS I: DERMOPATHY** ■ "Dermopathy" means "skin disease." Diabetic der-

mopathy is a type of dermopathy that occurs mostly on the shins, where some areas scar and develop dark pigment (hyperpigmentation). Other areas can atrophy (shrivel) slightly. Diabetic dermopathy can be linked to poorly controlled diabetes, but also to minor injuries and to aging.

986 MINOR SKIN PROBLEMS II: DIABETIC BULLAE ■

Diabetic bullae are blisters on the feet and legs caused by impaired healing resulting from poor blood-glucose control. Dermatologists see them frequently and treat them with antibiotics. Tight blood-glucose control is the best prevention and treatment.

987 MINOR SKIN PROBLEMS III: DIGITAL SCLEROSIS ■

Digital sclerosis is a thickening of the skin of the fingers. There may be callusing and less sensitivity. No definitive treatment exists, but researchers are working on the problem.

988 MINOR SKIN PROBLEMS IV: SCLERODERMA ■

Literally "hard skin," scleroderma is an abnormal thickening of the skin of the nape of the neck and upper back, making the area feel hard to the touch. It is caused by an overproduction of collagen and is treated symptomatically by applying prescription and nonprescription lotions and creams for dry skin.

989 MINOR SKIN PROBLEMS V: CAROTENIA ■

Carotenia is a yellowing of the skin, especially of the face, palms, and soles of the feet. It occurs mostly in fair-skinned patients.

In food faddists, carotenia is caused by eating enormous quantities of fruits or vegetables containing carotene, a red- or orange-pigmented phytochemical that is converted to vitamin A. But in people with diabetes, the cause is still a mystery.

Carotenia is harmless. It is not a sign of jaundice.

990 **MINOR SKIN PROBLEMS VI: ACANTHOSIS NIGRI-CANS** ■ Acanthosis nigricans is the medical term that describes "velvety" thick (hyperkeratosis), abnormally increased coloration (hyperpigmentation), warty overgrowths in areas of the body where there are skin folds—especially the neck, the groin, and the underarms. This condition is related to obesity. In most cases, the condition is benign, but should be checked at every doctor visit to make sure there have been no changes in these growths.

991 **MINOR SKIN PROBLEMS VII: NECROBIOSIS LIPOIDICA** ■ Necrobiosis lipoidica (NL) is a type of collagen degeneration. It is characterized by thickening of blood-vessel walls and the deposit of fat. While rare, NL occurs mostly in poorly controlled diabetics. Treatment consists of support stockings, elevation of the legs, and sometimes the application of topical steroids.

992 **MINOR SKIN PROBLEMS VIII: THOSE NASTY PAPER CUTS** ■ People with diabetes frequently have thin, dry skin and less than 20/20 vision, a perfect setup for paper cuts. Delayed healing means that these cuts are susceptible to further injury and infection.

If you don't want to see the doctor for a little paper cut, wash the area carefully and apply nonprescription triple antibiotic (bacitracin + neomycin + polymyxin B) ointment. Cover it with an adhesive bandage. Or ask your doctor for a prescription for Cleocin, a liquid antibiotic that penetrates the skin better than the antibiotic ointment.

993 **MINOR SKIN PROBLEMS IX: IMPAIRED HEALING** ■ Your doctor knows how "really delayed" the healing of your skin is. Most doctors urge their patients to contact them if there is no sign of healing in two days, or if their blood-glucose numbers skyrocket. Appropriate treatment depends on the type of skin injury or problem, its location, and its extent. Seriously delayed healing may call for stitches or even surgery.

Ladies and Gentlemen

994 **MAKE MINE MENOPAUSE** ■ Women's hormonal cycles affect their blood-glucose levels, and menopause does, too. Menopause is defined as the point when women have not had a menstrual period for twelve consecutive months. If you have diabetes, you can expect to enter menopause a bit sooner—but that could be anywhere between forty and seventy! A good indicator of the age when you might reach this eight-to-ten-year phase of life is the age your mother was when she reached menopause.

995 **MAMMOGRAMS ARE MANDATORY** ■ Premenopausal women with long-standing type 1 diabetes are particularly prone to an uncommon condition called "diabetic mastopathy": fibrous masses in the breast. The cause isn't fully understood, but doctors do know that women with diabetic mastopathy develop single or multiple firm or hard breast lumps that are not tender to the touch and that move easily under the skin. In order to reassure yourself that these recurring lumps are not malignant, women with diabetes should get mammograms and even fine-needle aspirations on a regular basis to keep track of these lumps and to spare themselves unnecessary surgical procedures—and worries.

996 **GENTLEMEN, CAN WE TALK?** ■ One of the least appealing aspects of diabetes in men is the problem of impaired blood flow to private parts, and the possible resulting impotence. Well-known diabetes educators June Biermann and Barbara Toohey have joined with diabetes expert Peter A. Lodewick to write a frank book about men's specific diabetic issues. Look for

The Diabetic Man: A Guide to Health and Success in All Areas of Your Life.

997 **LIFE AFTER *ANIMAL HOUSE* ■** The actor who played Flounder in the film *Animal House* is now spreading the gospel about diabetes. Stephen Furst and Stuart Pankin—from *Not Necessarily the News*—share their personal experiences with diabetes in the video, *Diabetes for Guys: A Guy Flick.* Definitely worth checking out!

998 **DON'T LIMIT YOURSELF TO NARROWLY DEFINED SEX ■** Physical contact is a basic human need, and needn't be limited to just the "working parts" you used in your youth. Very satisfying sex lives are possible for people whose diabetes have caused circulatory problems that affect erections or vaginal response. Rather than focusing on what's not working as you'd hopes, add empathy and foreplay and love and sharing to your experience. Remember, there's more than one way to achieve orgasm.

999 **WHAT IF IT'S NOT BAD, IT'S JUST DIFFERENT? ■** Ladies, if your man has diabetes, circulatory or nerve damage may necessitate patience and understanding that you haven't had to use before. Don't be critical or afraid of any delays or premature ejaculation. If he's suddenly reluctant, initiate—especially if that changes the pattern of interaction between you. Since he's got changes going on, your new creativity may be most welcome. Don't worry if he seems satisfied but doesn't ejaculate; he could be free to enjoy caresses and the sensual pleasures of extended foreplay—if he can get past any self-judgments or comparisons to real or imagined past powers.

1,000 **YOUR PARTNER'S SEXUAL RESPONSE ISN'T A JUDGMENT ON YOU ■** Please be clear about one thing: Any inability of your partner to achieve a firm erection or a lot of vaginal lubrication is *not* a judgment of your attractiveness or the state of your relationship. A man's erectile ability is physiologically dependent on blood flow and nerve response; a woman's capacity to lubricate may be affected by neuropathy. One of the best helps you can offer yourself and your partner is to remember that it's not about your adequacy to provide inspiration, it's about two people caring for each other's feelings and needs.

1,001 YOU AND YOUR DIABETES ARE A WORK IN PROGRESS ▪ This isn't Pollyanna talking.

Many improvements in diabetes care are on the horizon and should be available in the next five or ten years. (Just remember diabetes drugs ten years ago and you'll know what I mean.) Me? I'm looking forward to inhalable insulin!

You will make the greatest difference in what happens with your diabetes.

It only gets better from here!

Acknowledgments

THIS BOOK OWES so much to the help of many people, for whose time, interest, and enthusiasm I am indebted.

Special thanks go to Nao Esons, Claire Habermann, Annette Hard Lavine, Mischa Lieber, Michael L. McQuown, Elly Rumelt, Judith Rumelt, and prolific contributor Natalie Windsor.

I am also grateful to Robert A. Berger, M.D., Cathyann Corrado, D.P.M., Owen Cowitt, D.D.S., Myron Goldberg, M.D., Albert M. Harary, M.D., F.A.C.P., and especially Thomas C. Moore, M.D.

At Marlowe & Company, Matthew Lore, my editor, is a dream to work with and a brilliant diabetes resource. His assistant, Peter Jacoby, is wonderfully helpful and capable. Marlowe's managing editor, Vince Kunkemueller, was incredibly patient and understanding with this author who still prefers her typewriter. And Patty Park, Marlowe's publicist, is creative, hardworking, and marvelously effective.

This book would not exist without the unflagging support of Claudia Menza, my agent of many years and my friend for even longer.

Finally, my deepest thanks go to Harold Allen Lightman for his constant love and patience.